BY NIELS H. LAUERSEN, M.D.
*It's Your Body*


ALSO BY NIELS H. LAUERSEN, M.D., AND EILEEN STUKANE
*Listen to Your Body*

# *PMS*

## Premenstrual Syndrome and You: Next Month Can Be Different

### *Niels H. Lauersen, M.D.*
### *and Eileen Stukane*

**A FIRESIDE BOOK**
*Published by Simon & Schuster, Inc.*
**New York**

The illustrations on pages 139–51
are by Laurel Purinton Rand.

Copyright © 1983 by Niels H. Lauersen, M.D., and Eileen Stukane
All rights reserved
including the right of reproduction
in whole or in part in any form
A Fireside Book
Published by Simon & Schuster, Inc.
Simon & Schuster Building
Rockefeller Center
1230 Avenue of the Americas
New York, New York 10020
FIRESIDE and colophon are registered trademarks of Simon & Schuster, Inc.
Designed by Stanley S. Drate
Manufactured in the United States of America
Printed and bound by Fairfield Graphics
7 9 10 8 6
Library of Congress Cataloging in Publication Data
Lauersen, Niels.
PMS, premenstrual syndrome and you.
"A fireside book."
Bibliography: p.
Includes index.
1. Premenstrual syndrome. I. Stukane, Eileen.
II. Title.
RG165.L38   1983        618.1′72        83-11359
ISBN: 0-671-47242-9

# *Dedication*

To the silent sufferers of the past who never knew the cause of their troubles, to the pioneering women who dedicated themselves to the demystification of PMS, and to the women of tomorrow who, with knowledge, will free themselves from the syndrome.

# Acknowledgments

We owe a debt of gratitude to the many PMS sufferers who shared their experiences and taught us about the different faces of premenstrual syndrome. By expressing their honest feelings, these women inspired us to write a comprehensive handbook detailing the causes, symptoms, and especially, the treatment of PMS. Our appreciation is extended to each and every patient and friend who took the time to talk about the ways in which PMS affected their lives.

Special acknowledgment goes to our colleagues Dr. Zoë Graves and PMS counselor Paula Shara, for their skillful research and valuable suggestions.

Our sincere thanks to our loyal and talented assistant, Lori Leeds, who typed and helped to shape the final manuscript. Our gratitude also goes to Yvonne Brenner for transcribing the manuscript, and to Donna Almodovar for her secretarial help.

The original artwork was creatively produced by Laurel Purinton Rand, Ellen Felten, Lynne Cooper, and Judy Lief.

We have been fortunate to work with a number of expert professionals during the course of this book. These women and men shared information that took hard work and years of experience to acquire. We want to thank Hermien Lee for her professional advice on nutrition. This book's PMS Diet was created under her supervision. Fitness experts Olinda and Lazar Cedeno provided excellent exercises. Dr. Loren Fishman instructed us about yoga poses, and stress-management consultant Ron Shapiro shared his meditation techniques. These generous people broadened the dimensions of this book through their contributions.

Our appreciation also goes to our agents, Diana Price, Joyce Frommer, and Ellen Levine, for their advice and guidance.

We, in addition, extend our gratitude to our legal adviser, Richard Allan.

Many others have helped us in so many ways that we can do no more than thank them by listing their names: Ted May, Kathryn Park, Eileen Levine, Jayne De Point, Yanni Antonopoulos, Carol Ardman, and Leslie Lee.

We wish to thank Virginia Cassara, director of PMS Action in Madison, Wisconsin, for the knowledgeable direction she gave us during our investigation of PMS treatment and referral centers.

Finally, we extend our gratitude to Angela Miller, Jack Artenstein, and the supportive staff at Simon & Schuster, Inc., for their valuable assistance in the preparation of this book.

*Niels H. Lauersen, M.D.*
*Eileen Stukane*

# *Preface*

Years ago, when I first began practicing medicine, patients would tell me about the tranquilizers and painkillers that their doctors were prescribing for depression, mood swings, irritability, and headaches. I wondered why so many women were suffering symptoms that seemed to require these medications. After questioning women further, and investigating the published research, I came to discover that countless women were victims of cyclic symptoms, signs of premenstrual syndrome.

I soon began to realize the dilemma facing these women. PMS is a complex condition that was difficult for doctors to diagnose. Unlike most conditions, premenstrual syndrome had never been clearly defined by the medical establishment. The situation was a challenging one that most doctors avoided until it was researched and clarified by Dr. Katharina Dalton, the British physician who pioneered the diagnosis and treatment of PMS. I so admired Dr. Dalton's contribution to women's health care that, to show my appreciation of her important work, I was one of the first American doctors to endorse her book *Once a Month*.

My interest in premenstrual syndrome has brought me into contact with many sufferers who have made me understand that *recognition of the problem* is the essential step that must be taken if this condition is to be overcome. After recognition, a deep comprehension of the causes and treatments of PMS must follow. The frustration that I have often encountered in my own patients, I have also witnessed among the women I have met during my travels for my previous book, *Listen to Your Body*. Radio and television interviews have allowed me to talk to women I otherwise would not have known, and they have told me that PMS is a condition that they are only beginning to discover. They repeatedly ask for more information to relieve their suffering. Time after time I have heard the question: "Why didn't anyone help me understand PMS before?"

This book was written to answer that question. It is my hope that women will never again have to feel frustrated by a lack of knowledge about PMS. My co-author and I hope that this book will help women and all the men in their lives, whether they are mates or co-workers, to understand that premenstrual syndrome is a real condition caused by abnormal hormonal fluctuations in a women's body. PMS might be cured every time it occurs, if communication and modern treatment from doctors exist.

*PMS: Premenstrual Syndrome and You* is a handbook for the PMS sufferer and for the concerned symptom-free woman, but it is also a guide for men. Furthermore, it is my desire that the scientific explanations that are included will aid the many physicians who are beginning to recognize the monthly malady that women have experienced for generations.

—*Niels H. Lauersen,* M.D.
The Mount Sinai Medical Center
New York City
1983

# *Authors' Note*

In an effort to clarify the writing, when the authors refer to a woman's doctor, they use the male gender pronouns—he, his, him. The authors have given the book's hypothetical gynecologist a masculine identity to distinguish the doctor from the patient, who is always a woman and thus is referred to with female gender pronouns—she, hers, her. This doctor/patient gender identification must not be viewed as political or chauvinistic labeling; the distinction is made only to avoid confusion. The fact remains, however, that the overwhelming majority of OB/GYN specialists are men, a situation that, for the benefit of both patients and doctors, the authors hope will soon change. Many women are now entering into OB/GYN training programs and in the future a woman may have an opportunity to select a female or male doctor of her choice.

# Contents

# 1

# PMS—An Imaginary Disease?

"A Hymn to Him"

Women are irrational,
That's all there is to that!
Their heads are full of cotton,
   hay, and rags!
They're nothing but exasperating,
   irritating, vacillating, calculating,
   agitating, maddening, and infuriating hags!
Why can't a woman be more like a man?

Yes, why can't a woman be more like a man?
Men are so honest, so thoroughly square;
Eternally noble, historically fair;
Who, when you win, will always give your
   back a pat.
Why can't a woman be like that?

Why does every one do what the others do?
Can't a woman learn to use her head?
Why do they do everything their mothers do?
Why don't they grow up like their fathers
   instead?

*Why can't a woman take after a man?*
*Men are so pleasant, so easy to please;*
*Whenever you're with them, they're always*
    *at ease.*


*Q.—Would you be slighted if I didn't speak*
    *for hours?*
*A.—Of course not.*
*Q.—Would you be livid if I had a drink or two?*
*A.—Nonsense.*
*Q.—Would you be wounded if I never sent you*
    *flowers?*
*A.—Never!*
*Why can't a woman be like you?*


*One man in a million may shout a bit,*
*Now and then there's one with slight defects;*
*One, perhaps, whose truthfulness you doubt a bit.*
*But by and large we are a marvelous sex!*
*Why can't a woman behave like a man?*
*Men are so friendly, good-natured and kind,*
*A better companion you never will find.*


*Q.—If I were hours late for dinner would*
    *you bellow?*
*A.—Of course not.*
*Q.—If I forgot your silly birthday would*
    *you fuss?*
*A.—Nonsense.*
*Q.—Would you complain if I took out another*
    *fellow?*
*A.—Never!*
*Then why can't a woman be like us?*


*Why can't a woman be more like a man?*
*Men are so decent, such regular chaps.*
*Ready to help you through any mishaps.*
*Ready to buck you up whenever you are glum.*
*Why can't a woman be a chum?*

*Why is thinking something women never do?*
*Why is logic never even tried?*
*Straightening up their hair is all they*
    *ever do.*
*Why don't they straighten up the mess*
    *that's inside?*

*Why can't a woman be more like a man?*
*If I were a woman who'd been to a ball,*
*Been hailed as a princess by one and all;*
*Would I start weeping like a bathtub overflowing?*
*Carry on as if my home were in a tree?*
*Would I run off and never tell me where I'm*
    *going?*
*Why can't a woman be like me?*

—from the score of *My Fair Lady*\*

"A Hymn to Him" makes us smile at the "grandness" of the male ego and the dichotomy of the sexes, but what are we really laughing at? The way songwriters Alan Jay Lerner and Frederick Loewe describe women, they seem to belong to a different species than men. All those things about women weeping and being unpredictable and illogical . . . As if men were never that way! "A Hymn to Him" may be amusing and entertaining, but in their own talented ways, Lerner and Loewe have perpetuated ideas as old-fashioned as hoop skirts and calling menstruation "the curse."

Almost anywhere you look you can find women portrayed as if they are at one of two poles—either they are epitomes of perfection or cantankerous beasts. Literature is filled with these conflicting descriptions. Here, for instance, are classic examples in which women are presented so differently you might wonder whether you were reading about members of the same sex:

*The reason, firm, the temperate will,*
*Endurance, foresight, strength, and skill;*
*A perfect woman, nobly planned,*
*To warn, to comfort, and command.*
    —William Wordsworth
    "She Was a Phantom of Delight"

*A woman moved is like a fountain troubled,*
*Muddy, ill-seeming, thick, bereft of beauty.*
—William Shakespeare
*The Taming of the Shrew*

One or the other—either a woman is a faultless, wondrous being or she is an exasperating malcontent. These stereotyped portraits certainly have not helped the struggle for sexual equality, and, in fact, they almost seem designed to keep women suppressed.

It is no wonder that women have not wanted to discuss their health problems and private feelings with their male doctors. They might have been considered off-the-wall nuisances and dismissed. On the other hand, conferring with their doctors might not have occurred to patients who were trying to live up to society's image of the perfect woman—quiet and self-controlled, even when in pain. But sometimes suffering goes beyond tolerance.

It is heartbreaking to learn that when women finally speak up, doctors often tell them that their difficulties are "just nerves" or "all in their heads," and they prescribe tranquilizers to stop them from complaining. No woman should feel that she must endure her plight in silence or be looked upon as an irritant. Remember that Shakespeare's shrew is fictional. A woman who periodically experiences pain or depression must realize that her complaints are real. She actually may be a victim of premenstrual syndrome—PMS—a condition that some of the more progressive doctors have recently been willing to recognize and discuss with openness. Today, women can make their feelings known and take advantage of the medical profession's new interest in premenstrual syndrome. The condition can hardly be called "imaginary." It is a real problem, which doctors and patients should vow to overcome through proper therapy.

Still, many women might encounter physicians who have difficulty diagnosing PMS because its symptoms vary so widely. Sometimes even women themselves are not sure if they are sufferers because they are experiencing premenstrual syndrome in such mild forms. *The New York Times* recently reported that estimates of the total percentage of women who have premenstrual syndrome range from 20 to 95 percent. Most of the time, experts say *40 percent* of all women between fourteen and fifty years of age experience PMS. For the majority of women, symptoms are manageable, but it is estimated that 10 to 12 percent are so severely afflicted they cannot carry out their daily routines and must seek treatment.

PMS sufferers find that their symptoms begin anywhere from two to fourteen days before menstruation and last until the onset of, or a couple of days into, the bleeding. Mild symptoms, which women might not even know could be attributed to premenstrual syndrome, include appetite cravings—

longings for salt or sweets are the most common—a bloated feeling, abdominal swelling, constipation, frequent urination, breast tenderness, backache, forgetfulness, irritability, mood swings, and a general frustration with the tempo of daily life. On the other hand, women who have been diagnosed as having severe cases of premenstrual syndrome have complained of agitation, cyclic depressions, increased asthma attacks, episodes of epilepsy, migraine headaches, a loss of motor coordination, extreme emotional instability, and suicidal tendencies.

Often neither a woman nor her doctor will think of correlating a woman's clinical symptoms with her menstrual cycle, and time and again, this oversight accounts for not only inappropriate treatment but also a lack of information about the scope of PMS. While the most severe symptoms are indeed the most shocking, the majority of PMS sufferers only seem to be experiencing slight effects, and even women with the worst problems may have months when their conditions unexpectedly disappear.

While PMS is considered to be rooted in hormonal fluctuation, it also seems to be affected by a woman's emotions. Symptoms may vary from month to month as a woman reacts to the ups and downs of her family life, personal environment, working conditions, and not least of all, the stress that comes from living through each day.

It is my hope that by understanding what is known of the causes and symptoms of premenstrual syndrome women will be able to compensate for this very real, hormonally based, monthly malady. Awareness guarantees a route to health-improvement techniques and proper care from doctors. No one should have to suffer like Susan, a woman whose story unfolds below. This woman's life course was dramatically changed by premenstrual syndrome, and it was necessary to give her a pseudonym to protect her identity.

Susan's story is especially poignant because from the age of twelve to her present age, thirty, she had never heard about premenstrual syndrome and had thought that she was "crazy," that her emotional problems were untreatable. Most women do not experience psychologically devastating symptoms like Susan's. However, the events leading up to her discovery of PMS might help to enlighten all women, no matter how minor or major their symptoms might be.

### SUSAN'S STORY—"PMS DESTROYED MY MARRIAGE."

She began menstruating at age twelve, the same year that her parents decided to send her to a child psychologist. "Even I thought I was weird," says Susan, from her vantage point as a thirty-year-old woman. "I was extremely active, never sleeping at night. Usually I'd sit in my room and put together those model airplanes that come in kits. I never had any friends and my parents thought that a professional might teach me how to get along with my peers.

"Looking back, I feel that I was probably having hormonal problems even then, but what does a twelve-year-old know about hormones? I just did what my parents said and went to the psychologist."

A week after graduating from high school, Susan married Richard, a busy partner in his father's contracting business, and she went to work in a health food store. She had stopped seeing a therapist and life was comfortably routine most of the time. She emphasizes "most of the time," because she remembers the occasions when she felt like weeping without end. Back then she wanted to tell Richard what was bothering her, but how could she? Susan did not have a clue to the cause of her mournfulness; it was just that so often her whole life looked black.

However, once she conceived, those dismal days disappeared. Susan was indeed a serene madonna who felt blessed by the life within her body. She prayed for a girl and was ecstatic when Charlotte was born, but the postpartum depression that occurred when Charlotte was in the cradle never really went away.

When Susan was twenty-two, two years after her daughter's birth, she began to realize that her depressions followed a regular schedule. Richard was the first one to notice the pattern. He said that every few weeks he had to steel himself for a fight. She knew that the depressions felt like descents into an internal abyss. Susan would try to transcend her emotions but her despair would inevitably increase, frustration would build, and she would grow angry. She was at home with Charlotte all day, so she would tell herself, wait until Richard comes home, then I'll be able to talk this whole thing through.

But each time, when her husband walked through the door, she dissolved into streams of tears. She accused him of not loving her, of seeing another woman. One night she was screaming at him, pounding his chest with her fists, when in her hysteria she grabbed the collar of his shirt and ripped so hard that the buttons flew, pinging the toaster and the microwave oven. But before Susan could understand what she had done, she was knocked against the kitchen wall. Richard had smacked her across the face with the back of his hand. It was a forceful blow that cracked two teeth and dislocated her jaw. She had also bitten her tongue and blood was flowing from her mouth.

The bleeding instantly chastened them and Richard drove her straight to the emergency room of the nearest hospital. However, the next morning, he packed a suitcase and moved back with his parents. He was afraid he might hit her again because she was so uncontrollable when she was in a rage.

The separation lasted four months, and after many late-night talks and promises, Richard returned. They both resolved to try harder. After all, when

Susan was not out of control, she was a warm, loving person, a giving woman who enjoyed her husband and her child. At this point, Susan still had not heard about premenstrual syndrome, but she did think that her Jekyll-and-Hyde personality changes were somehow related to her periods. Her transformations seemed to overtake her about once a month, and they always occurred close to the time of her period.

A friend from the health food store advised Susan to try vitamin $B_6$, which was said to have an effect on the menstrual cycle. Susan was willing to try anything, but then she became pregnant with her second child. Just like the first time, the pregnancy was a welcome relief. She felt great. She never had a problem, not even with labor and natural childbirth.

Leslie was a fine, healthy baby girl, but once again, Susan was thrown into a severe postpartum depression and a few months later, the old depression and fits of temper began to occur once a month. The result was that her marriage again became unstable. Richard would leave for three months and come back for six. He did this twice but he would miss Susan and his daughters so much that the pain of parting would actually drive him home. Finally, he and Susan decided to find the solution that was eluding them, some way to save their marriage.

Susan was taking vitamin $B_6$, but it seemed to have no effect on her. She paid an internist $400 for a complete physical because she was sure she had a hormone imbalance. The doctor poked and prodded and, at the end of the visit, told her that there was no test for a hormone imbalance.

"If you're having your period, you have hormones, don't worry," said the doctor.

"There has to be more to it than that," said Susan. "Are my hormones high, low, what are they?"

"There isn't any more to say," he responded. "As far as I'm concerned, you have an anxiety disorder."

She refused to believe that no test existed, and she made an appointment with a gynecologist. He examined her and said, "You're healthy, and your hormones are fine." Then he said he would send her a bill.

Susan had charted her depressions and temper tantrums for months, and she knew that they occurred anywhere from two to five days before her period and lasted until she started to flow. Then she was fine. It was all too coincidental to be unimportant. She instinctively felt that her problem was physical, not mental, not an anxiety disorder, but the professionals were not giving her any answers and Richard lost his patience. He wanted them to go to a sex therapist.

In addition to the blues and the anger, Susan experienced a week of heightened sexual arousal. "Let's face it," says Susan with candor, "I was so horny I wanted to attack every man I saw on the street." She was making sexual demands of Richard that he could not fulfill. While he was trying to understand her, he was feeling dehumanized, as if he only existed as an object for her lust.

They began twice-weekly visits to a psychiatrist who specialized in sex therapy. Richard did not want to sleep with his wife anymore and his withdrawal from her increased her monthly fury. When she would scream, he would yell and storm out of the house. When he returned one time, Susan said, "You know this only happens once a month, you're forgetting your promise to understand." Richard admitted that he could not ignore the insults she hurled at him, the accusations of infidelity, and the general meanness in her voice. He was not able to forgive and forget the way she acted.

"I can't help myself," Susan would cry. "I wish I weren't a woman. I'd like to have everything taken out, a total hysterectomy. Take the ovaries, everything, so I don't have to go through this anymore."

Susan and Richard were emotionally drained, and during a session with the sex therapist, Richard said that he wanted to commit her to a mental hospital. Susan became livid. "How can you say I'm totally crazy when I'm upset only before my period?" she pleaded. Richard said that he did not care anymore. He had reached the limits of his understanding.

Susan reminded her husband and her therapist that she had consulted an internist and a gynecologist, and even though they had given her no satisfaction, she was willing to search further for the truth. She was sure that her menstrual cycle was involved. "Why don't you understand that that's just part of being a woman?" said the sex therapist. "You have other problems besides that."

She saw everyone as her enemy. No one appeared to be on her side, and there was no hope of saving her marriage. The hurts that she and Richard were inflicting on each other were too deep to mend. Richard moved away and initiated divorce proceedings.

It was only by chance that Susan later picked up a magazine from the rack at the supermarket checkout counter and saw an article about premenstrual syndrome (PMS). As she read about the personal experiences of other women with PMS, Susan realized that this was she, that she had PMS. Names of PMS clinics were listed in the article, and Susan was able to find help in her area. She underwent blood tests, and after a doctor diagnosed her as being a PMS sufferer, she was given special therapy. After a four-month period of experimenting with a therapeutic regime, she and her doctor arrived at the right treatment and Susan became a changed woman. The depressions and fits subsided and her daughters told her she was a "new mom." She sent the article that led to her cure to Richard, but he quickly mailed it back and wrote that he did not want to hear any more about "women's problems"; he had had it.

"Before I knew my problem had a name, PMS had destroyed my marriage," says Susan. "I want to do all I can to reach other women. My life was hell on earth because for so long no one told me what was wrong."

Many women have stories of their own, experiences that show how blind doctors have been to their problems. All too often, women like Susan have had to find the source of their troubles alone.

## WHY HAVE DOCTORS FAILED TO UNDERSTAND PMS?

A doctor who specializes in psychiatry, or for that matter, any field other than gynecology, may not think back to his early medical training about the female body. The possibility of premenstrual syndrome may never enter his sphere of thought, but since the condition has not been talked about for decades, he is not entirely to blame for the shortness of his memory. As recently as ten years ago, medical students were often taught that menstrual cramps and the symptoms of premenstrual syndrome were typical women's complaints without any basis in fact. They were made up, "all in a woman's head."

Historically, women have accepted the fact that they must bear monthly pain. They have even resigned themselves to possible death from motherhood because they are female. It is remarkable that it has been only in this century that the incidence of death during childbirth has diminished. In the nineteenth century, women who were about to give birth made out their wills beforehand. When a potentially fatal situation, such as childbirth once was, has only recently been reduced, it is not too surprising that the recognition of a condition that is not fatal has taken so long. In addition, another reason why doctors have probably steered away from premenstrual syndrome is because it is related to a woman's menstrual cycle, which human beings have so often perceived as mysterious and, by its very nature, powerful. And doctors, too, may have their judgments clouded by personal feelings about the monthly cycle. Menstruating women have been blamed or credited for everything from blight to harvests of plenty, from causing death to curing illness. Knowing this, menstruating women have not been anxious to complain.

Both women and doctors are just starting to overcome the time-honored myths about menstruation and to work together toward a mutual understanding of this natural, healthy, monthly cleansing of the uterus. The increase in health education throughout the country, which was inspired in part by the women's movement, has made certain facts about the female body impossible to ignore. The menstrual cycle must no longer be regarded in the way the Bible describes it, as "unclean":

> And if a woman have an issue of her blood many days out of the time of her separation, or if it run beyond the time of her separation; all the days of the issue of her uncleanness shall be as the days of separation: she shall be unclean.
> —Leviticus 15:25

In the Bible, a menstruating woman is also characterized as being "sick of her flowers." There is a certain irony in realizing that, rather than *during* menstruation, a woman may be seriously ill *before* menstruation, when she may suffer from premenstrual syndrome.

Finally, doctors are beginning to wonder enough about PMS to research medical literature and teach themselves about premenstrual problems. And it is amazing to realize that it was not in the last year or two that premenstrual syndrome was discovered but more than fifty years ago. In 1931, PMS was thoroughly described by Dr. Robert T. Frank of New York. He gave a meticulous explanation of the disorder in his now-famous thesis, "The Hormonal Causes of Premenstrual Tension." More than half a century ago, Dr. Frank's work should have been considered a breakthrough, but no one seemed to care that he had observed women suffer premenstrual disturbances as minor as fatigue and lack of concentration and as major as epilepticlike convulsions, bronchial asthma, and nervous tension severe enough to make them want to commit suicide. If Susan's doctors had only researched medical findings, she might have saved her marriage!

Yet it is not because women have been living in physical pain, frustration, or depression that physicians have begun to seek an understanding of premenstrual syndrome, nor is it because families have split up or women have committed suicide. The real impetus to everyone's sudden, consuming interest in premenstrual syndrome is *murder,* with PMS as a legal defense. Now that the lawyers have put premenstrual syndrome in the news, the doctors are willing to listen—they realize they have to.

## WHY DID IT TAKE MURDER TO CONVINCE THEM?

Suddenly everyone is talking about the syndrome that allows women to kill. U.S. reporters stunned the public with the news that the British courts had reduced two murder charges to manslaughter because the accused murderers, two women, had been shown to have had "diminished responsibility" due to PMS. The nationwide coverage was amazing, especially considering that before it appeared with such frequency in the media PMS was dismissed by most doctors as an ignorable condition, and many women had never even heard of it. Only researchers seem to have realized the extent of the problem.

Important findings about the distressing symptoms of PMS, and in fact the term "premenstrual syndrome," sprang from the efforts of two English physicians, Dr. Katharina Dalton and Dr. Raymond Greene, who in 1953 published the first PMS paper in British medical literature. One has to wonder why it took the sad loss of two lives to publicize a syndrome that had been investigated and analyzed for decades, a syndrome that could have been treated years ago. After all, at the time the news of the murder trials broke, it was fifty years after Dr. Frank's original findings and almost thirty years since Drs. Dalton and Greene had written their first paper on the subject. But obviously PMS had—or was given—a new wrinkle.

It almost seems as if the mostly male press corps, after years of hearing women say that they were equal to men, was anxious to expose a feminine flaw, a uniquely female condition that might make women emotionally uncontrollable and therefore unfit as decision makers. In the marketplace, where they are just beginning to gain positions of power, women feared that the misconstrued news about PMS might be used against them.

Recognition of premenstrual syndrome should have happened years earlier. Finally it was occurring, but in an incredibly backward manner. The shocking headlines obscured the real issue—the failure of doctors to diagnose and treat the condition. Also, feminists who had consistently denied the existence of PMS were put in the awkward position of commenting on the condition after it had been sensationalized. Women were said to have murdered due to PMS; how did other women feel about this? What about the effects of premenstrual syndrome? Maybe women really were the "weaker sex"!

A woman who has endometriosis or a tubal infection, two ailments a man can never experience, usually does not feel that her equality has been diminished by her feminine conditions. In the same way, she should not think that she is an inferior person if she suffers from premenstrual syndrome. Women who sense that they have PMS should acknowledge their symptoms, seek relief, and clearly regard it as a medical disorder. Had reporters more thoroughly presented the methods the courts had used to reach their decisions to accept PMS as a legal defense, the public might have realized that a great deal of medical research was involved. And PMS was considered to be *one* of the mitigating factors in the crimes, not some weird disease that would turn a normal, law-abiding woman into a homicidal maniac overnight.

Dr. Dalton herself has stated that a woman cannot merely say that she was premenstrual at the time she committed a crime, and be excused. "Evidence must be produced to show that the symptoms recur regularly each month, and that treatment is likely to be successful and ensure that she will not repeat the offense," writes Dr. Dalton, for it was she who was called in to diagnose the two criminal women.

## THE MURDER CASES

The first case centered on **Sandie Smith,** a thirty-year old barmaid from East London. Ms. Smith already had a record of about thirty convictions for disruptive behavior before she stabbed another barmaid to death in May

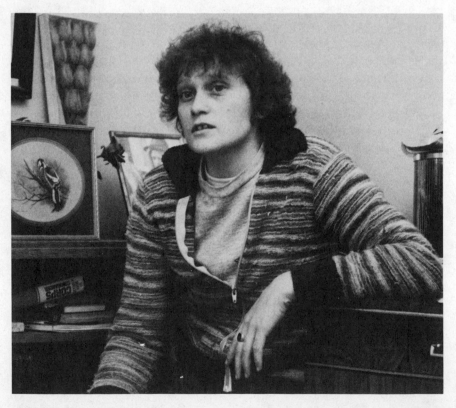

PMS victim Sandie Smith, who stabbed a barmaid to death, was freed on probation because of severe PMS symptoms. (Photographed by Terence Spencer. Reproduced by permission from PEOPLE Weekly/© 1982 Time Inc.)

1979. During Ms. Smith's murder trial, Dr. Dalton visited her in prison, and based on daily calendar notations that she asked Sandie Smith to keep, Dr. Dalton was able to diagnose PMS. However, Dr. Dalton continued to observe Ms. Smith for a year. Dr. Dalton kept daily behavior records that included notes on physical symptoms. She conducted physical examinations and ordered hormone analysis tests before and after Ms. Smith's progesterone treatment.

In May 1980, after evaluating Ms. Smith for a year, Dr. Dalton reported to the court that Sandie Smith's violent behavior could be controlled by daily injections of 100 milligrams of natural progesterone. Based on Dr. Dalton's conclusions after her year-long study of Ms. Smith, the woman was released on probation and ordered to receive daily injections from the district nursing service.

The accuracy of Dr. Dalton's careful diagnosis of PMS as a factor in Ms. Smith's behavior became apparent in October 1980, when Ms. Smith did not receive any injections for four days. With the absence of medication, Sandie Smith threw a brick through a window. She reported herself to the police and was released in custody, once again under orders to be treated for premenstrual syndrome. However, when Sandie's dosage was lowered and she was put on four injections a week, supplemented by suppositories, she tried to slash her wrists and, in an unrelated incident, threatened a police officer with a knife. She was convicted of intent to kill and carrying a weapon, but was released on probation with daily progesterone at the higher dosage required.

In the second case, **Christine English,** a thirty-seven-year-old woman with no history of violence or criminal behavior, was accused of killing her lover. What led a civilized woman to commit such a wild act of aggression? An explanation evolved from her medical history. After giving birth in 1963, Ms. English suffered a severe postpartum depression and this fact became crucial to her defense. As for her relationship with the man she was charged with murdering, it was always a stormy one.

In 1976, four years after her divorce in 1972, Ms. English met the man who became her lover for the next four years. He was an alcoholic who was easily provoked when he was drunk. The fight that led to his death was their last, but not their first, argument.

That night in December 1980, they were at odds over whether he was romantically involved with another woman. He ended the quarrel by bolting from the house. Ms. English waited a while and then went after him. She knew she had only to search the pubs and she would find him. When she caught up with him, they fought some more and drove to another pub. Ms. English was not drinking, but her lover was sinking deeper and deeper into an alcoholic stupor. The evening was a waking nightmare in which they were

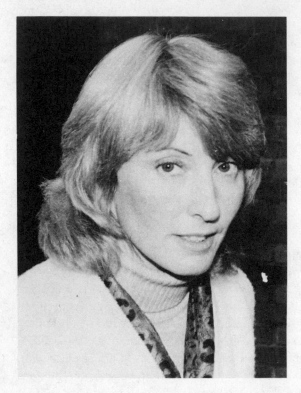

Christine English, who killed her lover with a car, had her murder charge reduced because of severe PMS. (Reproduced by permission from Richard Goss, director of Anglia Press Agency Limited, Colchester, England.)

shouting at each other, driving from pub to pub, and he was drinking. Finally, he asked her to take him home. She refused and drove away, leaving him in the exhaust fumes.

Then Ms. English had a change of heart. Perhaps she had a guilty twinge or maybe she wanted to make amends. At any rate, she turned the car around and returned to the spot where she had left the man. When she saw him, though, she lost control of herself, aimed the car right at him, and pinned him between her car and the lamppost. Shortly thereafter, he died from his injuries.

Her arrest was immediate. Ms. English was in a highly agitated state when she was accused of causing bodily harm (a charge that was later changed to murder with a deadly weapon, her car). Following a few hours at the police station, dawn approached and Ms. English began menstruating.

This time, Dr. Dalton and two psychiatrists were asked to examine the woman, and the importance of her postpartum depression was made known.

Dr. Dalton informed the court that about 90 percent of women who experience postpartum depression become PMS sufferers. (In "Susan's Story," it is interesting to note that postpartum depression also preceded PMS.) Dr. Dalton also reported that if women with PMS go for long intervals without food, they can become hypoglycemic, get a rush of adrenalin, and grow enraged. Christine had not had any sustenance for some time prior to crashing her car into her lover, and Dr. Dalton linked her rage and violence to an adrenalin rush from PMS-connected hypoglycemia. The defense also called another medical witness, who testified that Ms. English had suffered extreme premenstrual syndrome since 1966. All told, the evidence was strong enough to convince the judge that Ms. English had committed the crime under "wholly exceptional circumstances."

The PMS, the angry lover, and the fact that Ms. English was at the time in control of a lethal weapon, her car—all these facts led to the court's decision to reduce her charge to manslaughter on the grounds of "diminished responsibility" due to PMS. Dr. Dalton emphasized at the time that premenstrual syndrome was only one of the group of circumstances to be considered.

In order to be deemed PMS sufferers, Ms. Smith and Ms. English were scrupulously evaluated by doctors. The women had to be specially observed and it had to be positively shown that their behavior followed cyclic patterns that responded to natural progesterone treatments. It must also be remembered that witnesses for both the prosecution and the defense were heard in court. The women's charges were carefully considered, particularly because everyone connected with the cases knew that historical decisions were at stake.

However, the British actions do not mean that from now on lawyers will be able to plead "premenstrual syndrome" as an easy form of defense for a female client. PMS is a physical disorder that takes months to evaluate, and a woman who declares PMS as a defense for a crime must be shown to have cyclic symptoms that can be altered by therapy with natural progesterone.

So far, there has been only one case in the United States in which a lawyer has cited PMS. A Brooklyn woman, Shirley Santos, was charged with assault in the beating of her four-year-old daughter in December 1981, and her lawyer, Stephanie Benson, contended that the charges should be dropped because her client was suffering the effects of premenstrual syndrome. Ms. Benson is reported as saying, "When I saw my client in court she kept saying, 'I didn't mean to hurt her, I didn't mean to hurt her; I just got my period.' " Eventually, however, Ms. Santos pleaded guilty to a reduced charge of harrassment, and her premenstrual syndrome was never medically confirmed.

Since the greatest awareness of premenstrual syndrome has emerged from these criminal cases, the condition has been presented in its most extreme forms, and it is disturbing to consider that in everyday life PMS may be blamed for irresponsible behavior. Premenstrual syndrome is a real, hormonally based condition about which women should be informed so that as patients they may press their doctors to initiate treatment.

*PMS: Premenstrual Syndrome and You* aims to right the wrongful image of a PMS-crazed female who is emotionally out of control. Most women who experience symptoms of premenstrual syndrome are in physical discomfort, and although they may also be depressed or irritable, they have not lost their faculties.

In a recent *Glamour* survey of over 600 women, 71 percent said they did not believe that courts should accept PMS as a medical condition that produces violent behavior in women. However, 64 percent of the women reported that they suffered from premenstrual syndrome, and 38 percent revealed that their PMS was severe enough to disrupt their daily activities.

While it is most unfortunate that premenstrual syndrome has gained notoriety from acts of violence, it is helpful to have the condition openly discussed and recognized. The issue of whether PMS should be used as a legal defense cannot be resolved within the pages of this health guide. However, for the purposes of this book, the fact that in the *Glamour* survey 64 percent of the women knew enough about PMS to acknowledge that they were sufferers is promising. Women themselves can take advantage of PMS publicity to encourage their doctors to regard the condition with seriousness. When patients and doctors share a complete understanding and knowledge of premenstrual syndrome, women will be able to ask for, and receive, special attention and individualized treatment. Also, if the symptoms of PMS could be demystified and conquered, women might achieve the equality with men they deserve.

## DO MEN HAVE CYCLES TOO?

Women's cycles are clearly influenced by hormones. Men's biological rhythms are probably controlled by hormones too, but in a much less obvious way. However, in situations where testosterone, the male hormone, appears in excess or is totally absent, there are definite personality changes in men.

For example, it has been documented that men with more than one Y chromosome, "super males," as they are occasionally called, are often extremely aggressive and more prone to violence and dangerous criminal behavior. On the other hand, a man whose testosterone production has been stopped through castration or disease becomes docile and calm.

Centuries ago, castrated men, eunuchs as they are called, watched over the harems of mighty Roman emperors. The eunuchs, who were gentle with the women, had no sex drive and were able to serve as loyal guards. Sometimes the eunuchs were second- or third-born sons of ruling-class Roman families who early in their lives had undergone castration to prevent them from becoming rivals to the power of the firstborns.

It is important to good health that men, as well as women, recognize the significance of their hormones and pay attention to their patterns, because something curious is going on. Even though men do not have monthly hormonal fluctuations, they still report that they feel cyclic changes. And definitely in the overall picture of the life cycle, their feelings have been proved right.

In a ten-year study that became the basis for Gail Sheehy's book *Passages,** Dr. Daniel J. Levinson of Yale University School of Medicine analyzed the life cycle of a man. At the conclusion of his research effort, he was able to say that a man's life can consistently be divided into four phases, or "seasons," as he calls them. In his book *The Seasons of a Man's Life,* Dr. Levinson describes the "mid-life transition" that a man usually experiences between ages forty and forty-five. This transition is a crisis time for most men, and Dr. Levinson describes male behavior with an understanding that others should have when they write about the actions of premenstrual women.

"Because a man in this crisis is often somewhat irrational, others may regard him as 'upset' or 'sick.' In most cases, he is not," writes Dr. Levinson. "The man himself and those who care about him should recognize that he is in a normal developmental period and is working on normal mid-life tasks."†

Men have life, monthly, and daily patterns that are not judged harshly. And without being fully aware of it, men may be reacting both psychologically and physiologically to women's menstrual cycles.

In an Australian study, the basal body temperatures (BBTs) of women were simultaneously charted with the daily temperatures of their mates. Many of the men showed temperature elevations in the middle of the month, when the women's temperatures were also rising. The women's temperatures were going up because they were ovulating, but there was no physiological reason for the men's temperatures to climb. However, temperature comparability was a sign of overall compatibility. The study found that a woman's and man's temperature cycles were more closely in synch when the two were

---

*Gail Sheehy, *Passages* (New York: Dutton, 1976; paperback, New York: Bantam, 1977).
†Daniel J. Levinson et al., *The Seasons of a Man's Life* (New York: Ballantine, 1979), p. 199.

living together in harmony. There were few temperature correlations among women and men who were involved in troublesome relationships.

A man's identification with a woman and her cycles can become so strong that when she is pregnant he can actually take on certain symptoms of expectant motherhood. This "male pregnancy" phenomenon is called the Couvade Syndrome. From the French verb *couver,* which means to brood or to hatch, *couvade* was the term anthropologists used to describe the rituals that they saw expectant fathers in primitive tribes performing. For instance, while their wives were giving birth, men belonging to the Chaorati tribe in South America were seen mimicking the motions of labor and delivery and then resting in their hammocks for a few days. Today the Couvade Syndrome still describes the male imitation of pregnancy.

Research has shown that between ten to thirty percent of expectant fathers experience pregnancy symptoms that include everything from appetite cravings, weight gain, bloating, nausea, and vomiting to toothaches. One future father, suffering through nine months of indigestion during his wife's pregnancy, always had a bottle of Maalox at hand. After his wife gave birth to a healthy baby boy, his need for an antacid vanished with his anxiety. He was fine, but there are men who continue to suffer through postpartum depressions, either along with their wives, or by themselves while their mates show no signs of the blues.

Men, like women, also talk about being affected by outside forces such as the moon and the weather. The old myth that the moon makes men insane and sex-crazed still holds true. And during summer's heat, when the city streets are like steambaths, the crime rate soars. But whether the phases of the moon or the hot, humid days are to blame when men become emotionally unstable and lose control, there is far more chance that violence will erupt from them rather than from women. Men commit *90 percent* of the violent crimes. Although two British women became killers, they can hardly be called typical. Women do not make themselves battered wives, nor do they populate the prisons. And contrary to popular belief, there are more suicides among men than women. When it comes to self-inflicted pain and attempted suicides, men take the lead.

## PMS—YESTERDAY, TODAY, TOMORROW

For so long it has seemed that women have not been allowed to say what they are physically feeling and have not been taken seriously by their doctors. Women became so accustomed to hearing that their symptoms were "imaginary," they really thought they were fantasizing discomforts. Before women could ask to be treated for premenstrual problems, they first had to convince themselves that they were not "crazy" to think they were in distress. And sadly, women often were not able to make themselves believe the truth, that their suffering was real.

It is unfortunate that the reality of premenstrual syndrome was brought to everyone's attention through the sensational headlines about the British murder trials. However, the bright side of the surprising news is that premenstrual syndrome is now being seriously discussed among researchers, doctors, and women. Today, anyone who calls a woman "crazy" for admitting to premenstrual problems is considered unenlightened.

Actually, the interest that has arisen over PMS is reminiscent of the fervor that followed the public's awareness of hypoglycemia a few years ago. At that time, people debated whether hypoglycemia, a condition resulting from low blood sugar, was real, whether the information about the condition had been blown out of proportion, whether appropriate treatments existed. Today the controversy is no more; hypoglycemia is a medically accepted physiological disorder.

The furor over hypoglycemia subsided with information. Knowledge, which killed the controversy over hypoglycemia, will do the same thing for premenstrual syndrome. This book aims to break the silence that generations of women have kept while they suffered. As premenstrual syndrome is demystified and women take time to share their knowledge with each other, PMS will finally gain its rightful status as a medically recognized, treatable disorder.

# 2

# Revival of an Ancient Problem

The television specials devoted to premenstrual syndrome, the probing articles in glossy magazines, the newspaper reporters' interviews with doctors and PMS sufferers have turned PMS into a media event. The condition has been "introduced" as if it were a new discovery when in actuality, millennia ago, premenstrual syndrome probably affected primitive women.

PMS is an ancient problem that has suffered from a lack of recognition even though, throughout the twentieth century, for more than fifty years in fact, many scientific researchers—endocrinologists, gynecologists, and psychiatrists—have persistently studied and extensively reported its existence. It seems clear that the syndrome has been trapped under the taboo, the "curse" of menstruation.

The advancement of women's health needed the women's movement of the late sixties and early seventies to demand an end to all mysteries about the workings of the female body. Since then, many women have struggled to lift the "curse" of menstruation by educating themselves, as well as other women and men, about what a menstrual period really is—a natural monthly cleansing of the uterus.

Today most people know that menstruation is a normal, healthy process, not a disease or a sign of supernatural powers, but elements of old mysteries still linger. Why else would premenstrual syndrome be news? Why has it taken so much time for the condition to gain—and it still has not completely gained—medical acceptance? It seems as though the strangeness that was attached to menstruation has merely been passed on to PMS. Premenstrual syndrome is afflicted with the myths of menstruation, which are the source of religious beliefs and ritualistic acts that are older than the Great Pyramids.

One can understand how menstruation might have *originally* been considered a weird or magical event. Imagine primitive man watching primitive woman bleed for five days without dying. He must have been totally awed and frightened. And there probably wasn't any connection made to the fact that the reason a lot of the tribeswomen weren't bleeding was because they were constantly pregnant or breast-feeding. But then one has to wonder if all those primitives didn't notice that the animals bled too, at least when they were in heat.

Anyway, civilization progressed, but not the facts about menstruation. It seems logical that the word "menstruation" would come from the Latin word "mens" meaning "month," until you realize that "month" is a derivation of "moon" and that in Greek "moon" is "mene." The ancients were still identifying the monthly cycle as something cosmically controlled, like the phases of the moon. The interpretations of menstruation are mind-boggling.

A number of religions, which remain with us today, viewed—and sometimes still view—this very healthy and natural occurrence as repugnant. When Moslem women are menstruating they are not allowed to enter mosques. Women of Greek Orthodox faith, early in this century, were forbidden communion during their menstrual periods. At one time in the Catholic church's history, intercourse during menstruation was a sin. Even though menstruation gives a woman a wondrous internal cleansing, in the Orthodox Jewish faith a woman's "clean" days are *after* her period, when she is immersed in a purifying bath.

Cultural mores have also evolved from mistaken beliefs about menstruation and the omnipotence of menstruating women. There was a time when French and German women were barred from their countries' wineries and breweries because belief ran high that while they were menstruating, the women might sour the wine or beer. In *The Second Sex,*\* Simone de Beauvoir explains how in France a menstruating woman is known to have a bad effect on the curing of bacon, the fermentation of cider, and the refining of sugar. The myths in the Far East have prevented women from harvesting the rice paddies for fear that their menstruations would affect crop production, and the cattle in South Africa might still be kept away from menstruating women who might curdle the cow's milk. From country to country, menstruation has been considered a "curse." Premenstrual syndrome, being con-

\*Simone de Beauvoir, *The Second Sex* (New York: Knopf, 1952).

nected to menstruation, suffers the same, negative image, and with the British murder trials there is bound to be future folklore about PMS too.

Until recently, the most famous case of premenstrual syndrome probably belonged to Queen Victoria. In her book *Once a Month*,* Dr. Katharina Dalton cites the relationship of the eighteen-year-old queen to Prince Albert, her husband. Albert, a very rational man, could not find the logic in Victoria's unpredictable, emotional outbursts. She would hurl objects and scream at him, and no matter what he did—shouted, kept quiet—he was wrong. Only Victoria's pregnancies gave him spells of serenity, and he looked forward to them because pregnancy, at least, he understood.

Men have not comprehended the turmoil that can ensue within women during their premenstrual days, and women, since doctors have told them that they're physically fine, have not connected personally disturbing, out-of-control times to their upcoming menstruations.

It may be true, however, that today's women have greater opportunity to become aware of premenstrual syndrome because they are postponing childbearing. Modern contraceptive techniques have safely enabled women to have children later in life. This delay of motherhood is a departure from the traditional past, when women gave birth for the first time during their late teens or early twenties, and for the rest of their lives were frequently pregnant or breast-feeding and therefore infrequently menstruating. Living with fewer menstrual periods as they did, yesterday's women had hormonal levels that were more steady and they probably rarely suffered from PMS. Today, as women very often choose to have a career and to postpone motherhood until they are nearing or over thirty, they are experiencing more menstrual cycles and more menstrual problems than women encountered in the past.

Still, no matter what the menstrual myths or attitudes toward childbearing are, physicians had no reason to be uninformed about premenstrual syndrome. The condition had been extensively studied and reported in national as well as international journals, and papers on the subject had been regularly presented at medical seminars.

As mentioned in Chapter 1, more than fifty years ago PMS was methodically investigated and carefully described by Dr. Robert T. Frank of New York, although he, at the time, referred to premenstrual syndrome as "premenstrual tension." In 1931, Dr. Frank read his history-making paper, "The Hormonal Causes of Premenstrual Tension," at a meeting of the Section of Neurology and Psychiatry at the New York Academy of Medicine. (The paper was published shortly after his presentation in *Archives of Neurology and Psychiatry.)*

*Katharina Dalton, *Once a Month* (Pomona, Calif.: Hunter House, 1979).

One can imagine Dr. Frank, more than fifty years ago, reading from his introduction: "My attention has been increasingly directed to a large group of women who are handicapped by premenstrual disturbances of manifold nature. It is well-known that normal women suffer varying degrees of discomfort preceding the onset of menstruation. Employers of labor take cognizance of this fact and make provision for the temporary care of their employees. These minor disturbances include increased fatigability, irritability, lack of concentration and attacks of pain."

Dr. Frank went on to explain that he had encountered yet another group of women who complained of symptoms which kept them in bed for one or two days: "In this group, particularly, pain plays the predominant role." Then he reported on a third group: "There is still another class of patients in whom grave systemic disorders manifest themselves predominantly during the premenstrual period."

Women in the group that required bed rest probably were suffering from *dysmenorrhea,* the medical term for painful menstruation or menstrual cramps, a condition apart from premenstrual syndrome. Dr. Frank seems to have described many problems that come under the heading of menstrual distress: mild premenstrual syndrome, menstrual cramps, and severe premenstrual syndrome. Still, in writing a paper with the term "premenstrual tension" in the title, Dr. Frank brilliantly focused on a medical condition that needed, and continues to need, scientific recognition.

## PREMENSTRUAL SYNDROME OR PREMENSTRUAL TENSION?

Decades ago, scientists who were investigating problems associated with menstruation were struck by the constant appearance of what they labeled *premenstrual tension* (PMT), their umbrella term for depression, extreme fatigue, and irritability. However, as research in the field continued, it became clear that the "tension" evident during the premenstrual time was only part of what had to be called a syndrome—there were just too many other symptoms that consistently occurred prior to menstruation.

In addition to premenstrual tension, researchers discovered that symptoms women might experience anywhere from two to fourteen days before menstruation, and sometimes even a day or two after their menstrual flows began, included: food cravings, acne, leg heaviness, tiredness, mood swings, water retention, breast tenderness, backache, stomachache, joint aches, sore throat, flu, colds, headaches, dizziness, eye irritations, nervousness, sinusitis, crying spells, and an inability to concentrate. The definition of premenstrual tension had already expanded beyond depression, extreme fatigue, and irritability, to encompass: attempted suicide, asthma, epileptic seizures, migraine headaches, extreme anxiety, agitation, and angry, sometimes violent, behavior.

When researchers considered all the symptoms, they decided that they were really facing a multifaceted, recurrent syndrome. With all the facts before them, they settled on the term *premenstrual syndrome* (PMS) to describe the monthly symptoms that women experienced. Premenstrual tension, with all its debilitations, then became part of the larger, premenstrual syndrome.

But old habits are hard to change and many physicians still often refer to "premenstrual tension" when they mean the more comprehensive "premenstrual syndrome." There even seems to be a name preference based on geography. Physicians and scientists in Europe and the eastern United States are apt to use the term "premenstrual syndrome," while physicians and scientists on the West Coast of the United States will describe the syndrome as "premenstrual tension."

It is probably best for women who may be confused by the interchangeable terms to remember that if they are told they are suffering from premenstrual tension, they really have premenstrual syndrome. Throughout this book, premenstrual syndrome (PMS), the more inclusive label, is the term used to describe the many physical and psychological reactions a woman may have to her approaching menstrual period.

## HOW MANY WOMEN SUFFER FROM PMS?

Years ago, doctors may have considered that women with the severe symptoms of what was then known as PMT—depression, extreme fatigue, irritability, attempted suicide, asthma, epileptic seizures, migraine headaches, extreme anxiety, agitation, and angry, sometimes violent, behavior patterns—were the only women to be counted as PMS sufferers. Today, women and their physicians are aware that PMS includes all those just mentioned components of PMT, as well as milder symptoms such as food cravings, acne, leg heaviness, tiredness, mood swings, water retention, breast tenderness, backache, stomachache, joint aches, sore throat, flu, colds, headaches, dizziness, eye irritations, nervousness, sinusitis, crying spells, and an inability to concentrate. A woman who is a PMS sufferer may have one or a combination of ailments. The variety of ways in which the condition may manifest itself makes it difficult to get an exact count of the number of women afflicted. However, researchers have tried to compile statistics.

# PREMENSTRUAL SYNDROME

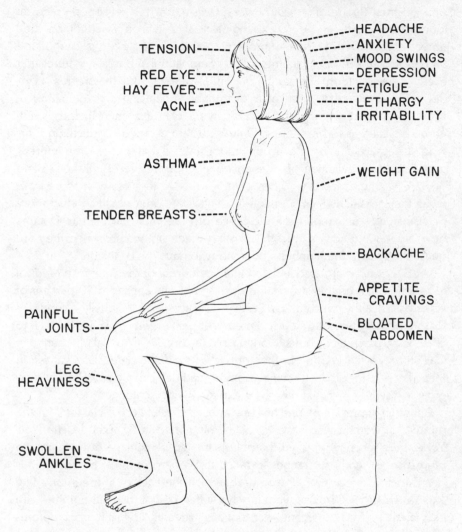

TENSION------

RED EYE------
HAY FEVER-----
ACNE------

ASTHMA-------

TENDER BREASTS------

PAINFUL
JOINTS----

LEG
HEAVINESS----

SWOLLEN
ANKLES----

------HEADACHE
------ANXIETY
------MOOD SWINGS
--------DEPRESSION
--------FATIGUE
--------LETHARGY
--------IRRITABILITY

------WEIGHT GAIN

------BACKACHE

APPETITE
CRAVINGS

BLOATED
ABDOMEN

*Typical Symptoms of PMS:* Some of the symptoms associated with PMS are indicated. A woman might suffer one or several of these symptoms at the same time. The symptoms usually occur anywhere from 2 to 14 days before the onset of the menstrual flow. (Reproduced from *Listen to Your Body,* Fireside/Simon & Schuster, Inc., 1982.)

In 1965, Drs. H. Sutherland and I. Stewart wrote "A Critical Analysis of the Premenstrual Syndrome," which was published in the prestigious medical journal *Lancet.* After analyzing existing medical reports on the condition, they arrived at their own definition of premenstrual syndrome. For Drs. Sutherland and Stewart, PMS was any combination of emotional or physical features that occurred cyclically in females before menstruation, and that regressed or disappeared toward the end of menstruation. Following their definition of PMS, the researchers found that 97 percent of the women in their study group qualified as PMS sufferers. Only 3 percent escaped classification! This type of statistical finding shows how important it is that someday an international standard definition of premenstrual syndrome be established. Right now, researchers may have different ideas of what they consider to be PMS when they are taking their counts. With a standard, they could conduct more precise studies and report the incidence of PMS more accurately. Doctors now use varying figures from the existing medical literature when they are questioned about the number of women who have the condition.

Dr. S. Leon Israel stated in 1938 in *The Journal of the American Medical Association* that premenstrual syndrome symptoms appear in 40 percent of otherwise healthy women. Dr. William Bickers and Maribelle Woods of Richmond, Virginia, who studied "premenstrual tension" in 1951, found it to occur in 36 percent of women working in a factory. Dr. Chunilal Mukherjee of Calcutta reported in 1954 in the *Journal of the Indian Medical Association* that 31.9 percent of 232 women whom he had determined had PMS had no organic disease that could otherwise explain their symptoms.

Although at present no one has been able to declare an official total for the number of women who have PMS, as mentioned in Chapter 1, *The New York Times* recently reported that the estimated percentage of women with premenstrual syndrome ranges from 20 to 95 percent. Most frequently it is heard that 40 percent of all women between the ages of fourteen and fifty experience PMS. Of those women who suffer, only a minimal number—an estimated 10 to 12 percent—are noticing severely debilitating symptoms which disrupt their lives.

Every woman has her own individual set of hormonal fluctuations. So by jotting down her physical and psychological changes on a calendar each month, a woman should, after three months, be able to determine whether she is regularly noting symptoms around the time of her menstruation. If she is, she is probably suffering from PMS.

## HOW SCIENTISTS HAVE TRIED TO TRACK
## DOWN THE CAUSES OF PMS

• *Hormonal Problems.* Back in 1931, when Dr. Frank reported the first fifteen cases of "premenstrual tension," he found high levels of estrogen in the blood and urine of his patients. He hypothesized that women who suffered from premenstrual tension probably did not properly excrete estrogen from their bodies, and high amounts of this female hormone remained in their bloodstreams.

As the estrogen in the blood circulated throughout a woman's body, it irritated her sympathetic nervous system. PMT symptoms surfaced, according to Dr. Frank, when the nervous system reacted to this irritation. So, very early in the discovery of PMS, the female hormones were considered important.

In 1938, Dr. S. Leon Israel of Mt. Sinai Hospital in New York also linked the female hormones to premenstrual tension, but he departed from Dr. Frank's theory. Dr. Israel performed D&Cs on women whom he had diagnosed as having premenstrual tension. He then scrutinized the tissue samples from the women's wombs under a microscope.

After his analysis, Dr. Israel, in a 1938 issue of *The Journal of the American Medical Association,* concluded that not all of the women had higher-than-normal levels of estrogen in their bloodstreams, but they did have persistent low concentrations of the female hormone progesterone. According to a microscopic finding, just before menstruation 75 percent of the women studied showed a very low level of progesterone but a normal or high estrogen level. Dr. Israel ascertained that the diminished progesterone was due to a deficient corpus luteum. The main producer of progesterone, the corpus luteum is a cell formation that develops within an ovary after ovulation. Dr. Israel's thesis, made almost fifty years ago, that PMS was caused by a low progesterone level in the face of a normal or high estrogen level, has been verified many times in recent years, and it is still the most accepted theory for the existence of this condition.

Knowing the cause of PMS, Dr. Israel tackled the condition in seven sufferers by injecting them with progesterone every other day during the last two weeks of their menstrual cycles. Five of the seven women were cured of all PMT symptoms and the other two women improved considerably. Thus, even back in the thirties, there was a clear indication that PMS was real, and due to an estrogen/progesterone imbalance that in indicated cases could be cured by progesterone injections. Dr. Israel had found the cause as well as the treatment of PMT. However, in the years that followed, researchers presented many other theories, in spite of Dr. Israel's excellent research. Hypotheses abounded, but the more researchers theorized, the more confused physicians became, and soon doctors started to doubt whether there really was a "premenstrual syndrome."

Other scientific theories about the causes of PMS:

• **A Toxin Takes Over.** Two Maryland physicians, Drs. E. J. Stieglitz and S. T. Kimble, in 1949 reported a phenomenon that they considered to be "premenstrual intoxication." They deduced that an unidentified chemical, a toxin in the body, caused mental, as well as physical, premenstrual symptoms. The doctors treated sixty-seven suffering women with ammonium nitrate, an acid diuretic, and reported that 91 percent of them were cured.

• **Water Retention.** In 1940, Drs. J. P. Greenhill and S. C. Freed introduced the idea that PMT was due to excessive salt and water retention. The salt in a woman's body was increased by the activity of her female hormones, the doctors reported, and salt in high supply caused body fluid to be retained. According to the doctors, when a woman became bloated, her nerve tissue and brain membrane swelled, and PMT symptoms occurred. The doctors treated fifteen women with oral doses of ammonium chloride, which lessens salt and body fluid, and all the women were relieved of their premenstrual problems.

In 1951, Dr. William Bickers and Maribelle Woods of Richmond, Virginia, corroborated the Greenhill/Freed theory that premenstrual tension was due to abnormal water retention, but Dr. Bickers and Ms. Woods were particularly interested in learning whether ammonium chloride was the most effective treatment. They found that a compound called pyrilamine 8 bromo theophyllinate relieved twenty-two women who were unaffected by ammonium chloride. No other researcher has verified this finding.

Water retention as a cause of PMT was also investigated by Dr. Chunilal Mukherjee in 1954, when he published his in-depth report, "Premenstrual Tension: A Critical Study of the Syndrome," in the *Journal of the Indian Medical Association*. Dr. Mukherjee found that twenty women who had never experienced premenstrual symptoms showed almost no weight gain before their menstrual periods, whereas twenty-five women with PMT gained an average of five pounds, in a range from two to sixteen pounds.

In his conclusion, Dr. Mukherjee attributed PMT to water retention and either an absence or a deficiency of the corpus luteum hormone progesterone. When water retention was the problem, Dr. Mukherjee was able to eliminate the symptoms with a low-salt diet and ammonium chloride. And when he deemed that the cause of a woman's PMS was hormonal, he achieved good results by administering progesterone.

• **The Vitamin B Theory.** Dr. Morton S. Biskind was the first researcher to suggest a connection between symptoms of PMS and a deficiency of vitamin B-complex. He did this as early as 1943! However, it was not until many years later that doctors—Dr. P. W. Adams in 1974 and Dr. D. P. Rose in 1978—confirmed a link between a lack of vitamin $B_6$ and the depressions some women experience when they are either suffering from PMS or taking birth control pills.

• *Hypoglycemia.* In 1925, six years before Dr. Frank's historic paper that coined the phrase "premenstrual tension," Drs. Okey and Robb reported that glucose tolerance curves were abnormal for women during menstruation and that women sometimes showed tendencies toward hypoglycemia, low blood sugar. Another observation of hypoglycemia came from Dr. S. Harris in 1944. In a report in the *Southern Medical Journal,* Dr. Harris noted that women frequently experience hunger, fatigue, nervousness, and sweating immediately prior to menstruation. He found a strong relationship between the symptoms of hypoglycemia and the functioning of the ovaries. In 1944 it was news to have a medical report mention that nervousness and cravings for sweets are marked in the premenstrual time.

Eight years later, in 1952, a large study of the relationship between hypoglycemia and PMT was conducted by a research team headed by Dr. J. H. Morton of New York. Dr. Morton and his colleagues administered glucose tolerance tests to 249 female inmates in the New York prison system. All of these women had reported symptoms of PMS, and their sugar tolerance tests showed hypoglycemic-type curves during premenstrual intervals. Almost twenty years later, in 1971, Dr. Y. Jung and a research team reported an overall incidence of hypoglycemia in 70 percent of a large female population.

Most women with PMS, whatever the cause might be, also suffer from hypoglycemic episodes after they eat large meals or sugary sweets. Indeed, a great number of women have found the symptoms of PMS are worse in the late morning and in the evening just before dinner—times when blood sugar levels are known to be low. Many of the PMS problems associated with hypoglycemia can be overcome by a low-sugar diet and frequent meals.

## UNDERSTANDING THE FACTS

Premenstrual syndrome has not been a completely ignored condition. Researchers have tackled PMS from many angles. They have analyzed symptoms and searched for a cause, but their conclusions have been so varied that doctors have been left to scratch their heads and ponder what the truth might be. Physicians have even looked with skepticism on the efforts of Dr. Katharina Dalton, one of the first doctors to recognize that a wide variety of symptoms might belong to *one* premenstrual condition.

Dr. Katharina Dalton is a British physician who in 1953 published the first paper in British medical literature on PMS. She wrote the paper with Dr. Raymond Greene, a noted endocrinologist who had also been working on premenstrual syndrome at the time. In fact, Drs. Dalton and Greene are credited with having created the term "premenstrual syndrome."

Dr. Dalton's experiences with her own period led her to suspect that premenstrual changes had far-ranging effects. She herself got a splitting migraine headache each month before her period. In 1953, when she was called in on the case of a woman who had asthmatic seizures each month just before she menstruated, Dr. Dalton started to consider linking different symptoms with the premenstrual condition. Another case of asthma turned up, followed by a woman with a monthly migraine. Drs. Dalton and Greene interviewed eighty-seven sufferers in order to write their first paper, and the rest, as they say, is medical history.

Drs. Dalton and Greene confirmed the estrogen/progesterone imbalance that Dr. Israel had written about in 1938. They also found, as Dr. Israel did, that PMS symptoms could be alleviated with progesterone treatments. Time and again, after the doctors administered progesterone, they  watched women shed their debilitating symptoms and assume control of their minds and bodies.

Dr. Dalton is now an acknowledged pioneer and authority in the field of premenstrual syndrome. She has been able to identify premenstrual changes as influences in criminal behavior, accidents, drug abuse, and death. Her work is applied to women in factories, schools, prisons, and hospitals, and there seems to be no one who has matched her dedication to the problem. As mentioned in Chapter 1, it was Dr. Dalton who was called in to diagnose Sandie Smith and Christine English, the defendants in the British murder trials that turned premenstrual syndrome into international news.

Now doctors have reason to research medical literature and gain an awareness of PMS from all the scientific papers that had previously caused confusion. Doctors can use the information gathered by past researchers to delve further into the causes of PMS. For, ironically, the scope of conclusions that arose from those many investigations actually helped the medical profession reach its current history-making decision—that *PMS is real.*

## A MODERN DESCRIPTION OF PMS

No two cases of premenstrual syndrome are the same. Every woman with PMS suffers her own set of symptoms, which need individualized treatment. However, with the many ways doctors have to diagnose and treat the condition come many chances to miss the right connections. Sometimes doctors may fail to pair symptoms with treatments that work. This problem of medical management occurs because doctors have never had comprehensive guidelines to follow in regard to PMS.

Premenstrual syndrome has definitely reached a time when it will be explored and defined with more exactness, but what happens in the interim? Women who need help today are visiting doctors who require more information to diagnose and treat their patients. What are doctors to do?

So far, a big effort to solve the doctors' dilemma has come from Dr. Guy E. Abraham, a former professor of obstetrics and gynecology at the U.C.L.A. School of Medicine, who joined the U.C.L.A Department of Obstetrics and Gynecology in 1971. Since Dr. Abraham has devoted his time and talent as a scientist to studying clinical problems in gynecologic endocrinology and nutrition, premenstrual syndrome falls perfectly into his sphere of interest.

Dr. Abraham fastidiously analyzed premenstrual syndrome, came to an understanding of its myriad symptoms, and defined it as precisely as possible. He divided the overall syndrome into four subgroups according to their symptoms. Then Dr. Abraham suggested specialized treatments for each subsyndrome that he had described. For the first time, someone had organized a way for doctors to diagnose the various forms of PMS.

Doctors learned about Dr. Abraham's simplification of premenstrual syndrome when his paper entitled "Premenstrual Tension" was published in *Current Problems in Obstetrics and Gynecology** in April 1981. In the editors' preface to this important paper, Drs. John M. Leventhal and Donald P. Goldstein, both highly reputed gynecologists, tell us that "Dr. Abraham has addressed one of the most common and least understood problems confronting the gynecologist. Premenstrual tension has all too often been considered an inevitable 'fate' of many menstruating women."

These two distinguished physicians continue to explain that this belief in "fate" has probably served to delay any understanding of PMS, which Dr. Abraham feels may affect as many as 12 million women in the United States. As the preface concludes, Drs. Leventhal and Goldstein announce that Dr. Abraham's systematic approach to this complex condition "provides the clinician with a significant understanding and allows for effective treatment of the woman who no longer needs to be left to her monthly premenstrual 'fate.' "

*Guy E. Abraham, "Premenstrual Tension," *Current Problems in Obstetrics and Gynecology* (Chicago: Year Book Medical Publishers, April 1981).

## ADOPTING THE NEW APPROACH

Dr. Abraham uses the term "premenstrual tension" to classify the condition that in this book is considered to be premenstrual syndrome. The references to his subsyndromes, therefore, bear the initials PMT, which here should be considered synonymous with PMS.

According to Dr. Abraham, premenstrual syndrome can be divided into the following four subgroups—PMT–A, PMT–H, PMT–C, and PMT–D—which are described below.

• **PMT–A.** Women would be diagnosed as having PMT–A when they mainly complain of anxiety, irritability, and nervous tension occurring as early as midcycle and intensifying as the cycle approaches menstruation. Sometimes women in this group may say that they also experience mild to moderate depression as their menstrual periods near. However, no matter how much the symptoms of PMT–A seem to grow worse as the cycle progresses, in the end menstruation brings relief.

According to Dr. Abraham, most women who have PMS would be classified in the PMT–A group. He feels that this subgroup includes the most commonly mentioned symptoms. Increased anxiety, hostility, and depression during the premenstrual time have frequently been documented in medical reports and Dr. Abraham concludes that this behavior becomes expressed when "the appropriate environmental stimuli" are present. These "stimuli" may be anything from family problems to on-the-job stress.

Women with PMT–A have been found to have hormonal imbalances occurring when estrogen is high in relation to progesterone during the last half of the menstrual cycle. In the case of such a hormonal imbalance, the natural approach to treating PMS may not be sufficient in all cases. A woman with PMT–A may need progesterone replacement in addition to the natural approach, both of which are explained in Chapter 5.

• **PMT–H.** Perhaps Dr. Abraham used the initial "H" here to signify "heaviness." Women who fall into the PMT–H category would experience premenstrual weight gain, abdominal bloating, tenderness around the abdomen and breasts, breast congestion, and occasional swelling of the face, legs, and arms. Usually less than a three-pound weight gain occurs premenstrually, but women with severe PMT–H may put on five or more pounds before their menstrual periods. Sometimes, as women get older, they have difficulty losing premenstrual weight, which should normally disappear with the onset of menstruation.

PMT–H appears in 60 to 66 percent of PMS sufferers and is often found along with symptoms of other subgroups. The problems of PMT–H stem from an increase in extracellular fluid, or, put more simply, water is retained outside the blood vessels. PMT–H is partly due to an increase in the body's salt concentration. A woman may be ingesting more salt than usual to calm a craving, or she may have an imbalance in the salt-retaining adrenal hormone, aldosterone. Whatever the reason, the resulting water retention brings on a feeling of heaviness.

• **PMT–C.** Women with PMT–C succumb to increased appetites and cravings for sweets, and then twenty to sixty minutes after they eat large amounts of refined carbohydrates and sugar they experience fainting spells, fatigue, palpitation, and headaches. Researchers have confirmed a positive correlation between this premenstrual craving for sweets and feelings of stress-related tension.

As Dr. Abraham explains in his analysis of this subgroup, the brain, which normally uses 20 percent of the body's total energy, demands even more energy when it is under stress. This extra energy must come from glucose, which the liver must produce from sugar. However, the liver needs nutrients, especially the B vitamins and magnesium, to break down sugar and turn it into glucose.

The process seems simple enough, but sometimes a woman does not have the B vitamins and magnesium that make the liver's sugar–glucose conversion possible. At this point, the brain sees to it that the necessary nutrients are supplied.

If the brain-under-stress does not get the energy-giving glucose it needs, it releases signals that trigger a woman's craving for sweets. A chocolate craving, for example, might be a sign of magnesium deficiency, since chocolate is rich in magnesium. A woman then responds by eating the nutrient-necessary foods.

After ovulation, in the last half of the menstrual cycle, cells bind insulin, and with an increased sugar intake, the overall insulin level in a woman's body climbs. This rise in insulin triggers hypoglycemia with its resulting PMT–C fainting, fatigue, palpitation, and headache.

PMT–C may be avoided if the brain is not stressed. It is important that women with PMT–C reduce their stress levels while they increase their intakes of vitamins and minerals. It takes great will power to refrain from the sweets that the brain-under-stress is signaling it needs, but even so, a woman should try to shy away from sweets and prevent the body process that brings on PMT–C. (Detailed methods for overcoming PMT–C are described in Chapter 5.)

• **PMT–D.** Premenstrual depression, withdrawal, thoughts of suicide, and suicide attempts are symptoms of PMT–D. Women in this subgroup also complain of lethargy, confusion, incoherence, and difficulty with verbalization. When PMT–D is severe, a woman may be too depressed to complain and she may need a friend who is attuned to her plight to bring her to a psychiatrist. In fact, statistics reveal that women with severe PMT–D are brought for professional help by friends more often than they seek care alone.

It is fortunate that friends intervene, because research has shown that the woman who does not complain is more likely to attempt, and succeed in committing, suicide than the woman with a combination of PMT–A and PMT–D who talks about her anxiety. Most of the time, however, PMT–D does follow the anxiousness and irritability of the PMT–A type. Dr. Abraham reports that "pure PMT–D may be present in less than three percent of PMT patients." And when pure PMT–D does occur, there seems to be a hormonal imbalance in which progesterone is especially high in relation to estrogen during the last half of the menstrual cycle. Dr. Abraham has suggested that a nutritional deficiency that lowers a woman's resistance to her stress and hormonal imbalance causes PMT–D to surface.

Dr. Abraham's detailed subdivision of premenstrual syndrome is extremely important for women and their doctors. It helps to promote an understanding of the complexity of PMS. It should also aid physicians in finding the best treatments for individual complaints.

## THE EVIDENCE IS UNDENIABLE

PMS cannot be dismissed as a fad occurring because two murder trials in England brought it to the world's attention. More than fifty years of scientific research have been devoted to tracking down the causes of this condition, and many years of investigation are still needed.

Professors in medical schools and postgraduate courses for doctors will hopefully soon begin to inform future and current physicians about the many medical findings that focus on PMS. With modern technology, particularly with the development of the radioimmunoassay, the testing technique that enables doctors to measure minute hormonal levels in the blood, researchers are better equipped to investigate a woman's delicate hormonal fluctuations. Interactions between the brain hormones and the ovarian hormones can become better understood. The complexity of all hormonal secretions can be confronted and simplified. The acceptance of PMS as a multifaceted condition, with each case individualized, should be a goal for all women and their doctors.

In the past, women have been hospitalized or treated with tranquilizers and other inappropriate medications when they have been suffering from premenstrual syndrome. Those myths about menstruation that opened this chapter must never again be used to hinder understanding of the menstrual cycle or its accompanying PMS. It is time to replace conjecture with scientific fact.

# 3

---

# PMS Is Real!

Eleanor splashed cold water on her face and composed herself in front of the ladies' room mirror. She had forsaken twenty-four fifth-graders in the midst of a history lesson because she had felt a flood of tears banking itself behind her eyes. It was an insuppressible flood. She was out of control.

Eleanor was a talented teacher, a figure of authority, a person who had never before shown emotion in front of her students. Yet she had fled the room in tears. The urge to weep, which she had experienced as strongly as if she had just heard tragic news of a loved one, had suddenly ruled.

"Get a grip," Eleanor said to her mirrored reflection, as she wondered what was happening to her. She had had spells of sobbing and weeping in the past, but they had never occurred in class. It was only two days after the ladies' room episode, when her period arrived, that she started to realize that an attack of tears took place almost every time she was due to menstruate.

Eleanor made an appointment with her doctor because she thought she might be having trouble with her hormones. After she explained everything that she could recall about her cyclic crying to him, the doctor examined her carefully. Later, in his consultation office, he cleared his throat and told her quite seriously, "I believe you have symptoms of premenstrual syndrome. There are various kinds of PMS and yours seems to be the A-type. This kind has anxiety, agitation, and mood swings predominating."

That explanation did not satisfy Eleanor. "You may have given my problem a name, but you haven't told me *why* I cry. What happens to me?" she asked, and, challenged by her direct gaze, her doctor tried his best to answer.

"I can see that you need more information. It might be difficult for you to understand, because sometimes we doctors don't fully understand," he said, "but PMS is a real, most probably hormonally based condition. I am going to ask you to mark down your daily symptoms on a calendar so that we have a clear indication of how and when you are suffering. I'll also order hormonal analyses of your blood samples, and together we'll both learn how to diagnose and treat your particular case."

As Eleanor finished telling the story of how she had discovered her PMS, I thought how fortunate she was to have an enlightened gynecologist.

## CONFUSION OVER THE CAUSES OF PMS

A growing number of doctors are intellectually aligned with Eleanor's physician. These progressive professionals recognize PMS as real and seek to educate themselves and their patients to its causes, symptoms, and treatments. There are many theories about the reasons for PMS. The most significant ones, those described in Chapter 2, have helped doctors understand premenstrual syndrome, but they've also opened the condition to question.

As theories on the causes of PMS have accrued, researchers have found more facts to investigate and less reason to reach agreement. Doctors have pointed to this complexity of causes and symptoms as grounds for the right either to dismiss PMS or to attribute it to "a woman's neurosis." However, by defining the condition as a woman's neurotic invention, doctors have subtly set back the demystification of the syndrome. Since women have, until recently, been reluctant to discuss premenstrual symptoms with their doctors, as patients they have also, albeit unwittingly, impeded the progress of research. Finally, though, the fog around the existing theories is beginning to lift and although there continues to be debate about the exact cause of PMS, most physicians are able to agree on one fact: namely, that premenstrual syndrome at some point hinges on the effect of hormonal fluctuation.

My personal belief is that PMS is triggered by hormonal irregularities in a woman's body. However, there is still some question as to which hormones are involved and what the imbalances might be. Dr. Leon Israel and Dr. Katharina Dalton each have indicated that most of the symptoms of premenstrual syndrome are caused by excessive estrogen and deficient progesterone levels. Although the high estrogen/low progesterone imbalance may occur in many patients, it is not the source of every woman's PMS. As pointed out in this chapter, other hormones and various mitigating factors are involved.

Each PMS sufferer is unique. Symptoms vary from woman to woman, and sometimes from month to month. A woman with PMS should be carefully interviewed as to the type and frequency of her symptoms. Hormonal analyses of her blood samples should also be conducted. After a detailed investigation into a woman's health history, her treatment should then be formulated. PMS treatment should always be individualized, specifically designed on a patient-by-patient basis. Although all the studies seem to produce different theories as to the causes of PMS, most findings can be traced back to the changing sensitivity of a woman's body at various times during her menstrual cycle. This sensitivity may be rooted in hormones, but it may not need hormonal treatment to be adjusted. It may be possible to eliminate a woman's symptoms by modifying her diet, vitamin, and exercise regimens, rather than by prescribing supplementary hormones.

Every woman, therefore, needs a deep understanding of her menstrual cycle in order to know why she might be experiencing symptoms of premenstrual syndrome. If she could visualize what normally happens during the course of her menstrual cycle, the time from one period to another when complex but wonderfully designed hormonal fluctuations occur in her body, a woman would instinctively recognize when something is wrong.

## THE EBB AND FLOW OF THE MENSTRUAL CYCLE

On the first day of a woman's period, one menstrual cycle has just ended and another is beginning. A woman has arrived at day one of a brand-new cycle.

A few days later, as the menstrual flow starts to diminish, the hypothalamus of the brain, which controls the menstrual cycle, sends a hormonal message—the Releasing Factor—to the pituitary gland. This message does not have to travel far, because the pituitary is located just below the hypothalamus.

When the pituitary receives the message, it releases the Follicle Stimulating Hormone—FSH—which travels through the blood to the ovaries, and then the action begins. The ovaries start to work and all the little follicles, the potential egg cells in the ovaries, begin to grow and produce the female hormone estrogen. A woman's skin may start to feel smoother as her estrogen builds.

As the estrogen increases, it sends a "slow down" message back to the pituitary. At about this time, a woman's breasts are becoming a little bigger and one of the follicles, for some unknown reason, is beginning to surpass the other egg cells in its development. That one egg cell, called the Graafian follicle or the follicle(egg)-of-the-month, bubbles out on the outside of the ovary. This bubble contains the egg that is destined for a trip to the womb.

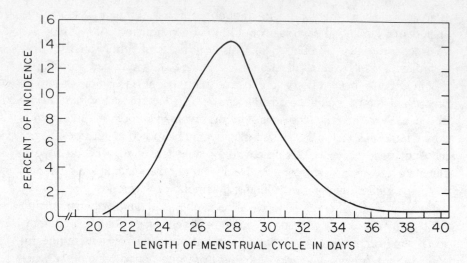

*Duration of the Menstrual Cycle:* The number of days from one menstruation to another varies anywhere from 21 days to, occasionally, more than 40 days. The average length, as seen in the illustration, is around 28 days. (Reproduced from *Listen to Your Body,* Fireside/Simon & Schuster, Inc., 1982.)

About thirteen or fourteen days into the cycle, the pituitary responds to the increased estrogen by sending out the Luteinizing Hormone—LH—and stopping the FSH. The LH makes the Graafian follicle burst and eject a mature egg cell—this release of the egg is *ovulation.* The egg then strikes out on a five- to seven-day journey inside the Fallopian tube to the womb.

The scar tissue that's left behind after the egg pops out becomes the *corpus luteum,* the producer of progesterone, the pregnancy hormone. Progesterone causes the lining of the uterus to change into a soft, spongy nest rich in blood vessels and glandular tissue that forms the perfect bed for the egg coming down the tube. The hormone also relaxes the uterus to give the egg a better chance to implant itself into the endometrium, the transformed uterine lining.

Estrogen and progesterone increase together after ovulation, as the LH drops off. However, there are a number of side effects that come from the surge of estrogen and progesterone during this last half of the menstrual cycle, and these are discussed in the section that follows.

Meanwhile, as the menstrual cycle nears an end, if the egg is fertilized and pregnancy occurs, estrogen and progesterone levels stay high. But if there is no fertilizatiuon, the brain does not get the stimulus it needs to maintain the corpus luteum. The corpus luteum disintegrates, progesterone and estrogen levels drop rapidly, and menstruation is triggered. The *endometrium*—the enriched spongy lining of the uterus—which is useless without pregnancy, leaves the body as menstrual blood. Then, once again, one menstrual cycle ends and another begins. A woman arrives at day one of a brand-new cycle.

It is important to mention, however, that most women do not have exact twenty-eight-day menstrual cycles. In fact, the time span of cycles for any given group of women can realistically be plotted on a Bell curve (*see* figure opposite). Some women have their periods in fewer than twenty-eight days, while others live with cycles that may take thirty, thirty-one, thirty-four, or more days from start to finish. Every woman usually knows what is "normal" for her, and she senses when "normal" goes haywire.

### THE KEY TO PMS—THE ESTROGEN/PROGESTERONE IMBALANCE

It is during the last half of the menstrual cycle, the fourteen days between ovulation and menstruation, that estrogen and progesterone first peak and

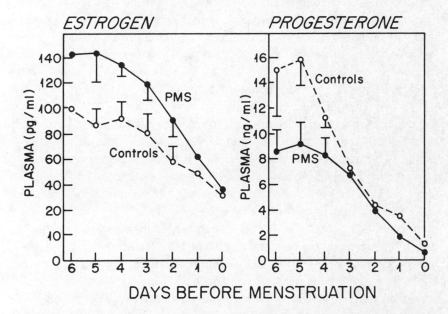

*Hormone Levels in Normal and PMS Patients Before Menstruation:* In women with severe PMS, which has anxiety and mood swings as two of its main symptoms, the premenstrual estrogen levels are higher and the progesterone levels lower, when comparisons are made with controls—women without PMS. (Reproduced from *Listen to Your Body,* Fireside/Simon & Schuster, Inc., 1982.)

then fall. If these two surging hormones lose their normally fine balance, they can become the key to premenstrual syndrome. Although each case of premenstrual syndrome is unique and mitigating factors may be contributing to symptoms, most often the source of PMS can be directly or indirectly linked to hormone-regulating mechanisms in a woman's body. There are theories that the condition might be related to the brain hormones, but in most cases, fluctuation of the ever mystifying female hormones is a much more likely cause.

However, before discussing how these hormones might make a calm woman feel like a coiled spring, there's good news. There is a positive side to the estrogen/progesterone rush after ovulation. Estrogen increases the blood supply to the endometrium, the uterine lining that progesterone is turning into a bed for fertilization. Estrogen also makes a woman's skin smooth and blemish-free. Besides being the architect of the endometrium, progesterone relaxes the womb, alters the cervical mucus so that it thickens and shields the uterus from infection, and can, in combination with estrogen, stimulate the sex drive. Just like a pregnant woman—who, living with an increase of estrogen and progesterone for nine months, often feels sexier—a woman who has a high amount of female hormones after ovulation sometimes responds more sexually too. When these hormones are in balance, women feel wonderful. When estrogen and progesterone are not in tune, when there's too much of one or too little of the other, all sorts of symptoms connected to premenstrual syndrome may arise.

Estrogen binds salt and salt binds water, so a high amount of estrogen can lead to water retention, an edema that can cause a swelling of body tissues in the stomach, breasts, legs, and even in the brain. Swelling in the brain is especially serious, because when the brain becomes bloated with extra fluid it expands. However, the brain, encased within the skull, can only expand as far as the skull permits. Then the nerve tissue that surrounds the brain feels the extreme pressure of the brain's expansion. It is believed that it is this pressure, this stretching of the brain membrane, that leads to headaches, irritability, inability to concentrate, migraines, seizure disorders, dizziness, and hypersensitivity to light, which are all symptoms of premenstrual syndrome. Not to be forgotten, the rest of a woman's body feels heavy and bloated too. A woman may experience an added pressure in her abdomen and bowel area, and she might have gas pains.

However, even if a woman has an excessive amount of estrogen, the widely held medical belief is that she will not show signs of PMS if she produces enough natural progesterone to counteract the effects of her abundant estrogen supply. A number of symptoms of premenstrual syndrome occur when there is too much estrogen in relation to progesterone.

There is, though, some question as to whether symptoms related to too little progesterone surface because there's an abundance of estrogen or a deficiency of progesterone. Dr. Katharina Dalton attributes certain PMS symptoms to a *lack* of progesterone, and she has successfully treated women with natural progesterone suppositories. Treatments will be covered in depth in Chapter 5.

The appearance of progesterone in the second half of the menstrual cycle may create a variety of symptoms. These symptoms will be more pronounced if there isn't just enough estrogen to balance the progesterone. There will be bladder pressure and bowel irritation from which gas and constipation may result. Progesterone is a Latin name that literally translated means "for (pro) gestation (gesterone)." This hormone "for gestation" is also called the pregnancy hormone or the hormone of the mother. Progesterone maintains pregnancy, but, whether or not a woman is pregnant, the hormone also is known to make certain symptoms appear.

During pregnancy, a woman may have ravenous food cravings due to elevated progesterone levels, and when progesterone is present in the last half of the menstrual cycle of a woman who is not pregnant, she may have similar cravings. She might long for sweets due to lowered blood sugar, and at the same time she may feel hot because her body temperature has risen. At this time, women may also develop acne, allergic reactions, and have little resistance to infection. In addition, too much progesterone can make a normally energetic woman feel incredibly fatigued. Physical symptoms can become so severe that they upset a woman's mental health.

## THE POWER OF THE BRAIN

It seems fairly certain that PMS must be due to the fluctuation of the female hormones estrogen and progesterone, but this fluctuation is initially orchestrated by brain hormones that—as we are learning—influence, and are influenced by, the way a woman responds to her personal environment.

Recently, one leader in the field of reproductive endocrinology, Dr. Sam S. C. Yen, chairman of the department of reproductive medicine, School of Medicine, University of California in San Diego, in association with Dr. Robert L. Reid, presented revolutionary ideas about PMS. The Reid/Yen report, which evaluated much of the existing knowledge about PMS, appeared in the prestigious *American Journal of Obstetrics and Gynecology*. Gynecologists around the world were able to read about PMS, a condition that these outstanding physicians called "a major clinical entity affecting a large segment of the female population."

Drs. Reid and Yen suggested a possible new source of PMS. They hypothesized that the syndrome was caused by events of the neuroendocrine system. "Neuroendocrine" is a word that has been created to define a combination of the nervous system and the endocrine, or hormonal, network in the body. The doctors referred to the way the hypothalamus and pituitary gland in the brain receive nerve-transmitting signals to release hormones that instigate endocrine activity in the ovaries and other parts of the body. Their new offering to science is that the nerve-transmitting signals in the brain come from the peptides alpha-melanocyte-stimulating-hormone (alpha–MSH) and beta-endorphin, and that the interaction between the hypothalamus and the pituitary is influenced by these peptides during the last half of the menstrual cycle. (Peptides are amino acid compounds that originate in the brain's neurointermediate lobe.)

The ebb and flow of the alpha-MSH and beta-endorphin may be responsible for shifts in a woman's mood and behavior as well as changes in her hormonal fluctuations. Estrogen, progesterone, prolactin, and vasopressin, a pituitary hormone that regulates blood pressure, may all be affected by the actions of the peptides. On the other hand, the scientists believe that external forces such as stress, unhappiness, travel, weight gain or loss, divorce, surgery, major life changes, or traumatic events may also influence the neuroendocrine system and, in turn, the menstrual cycle. In other words, outside forces may sometimes influence the peptides before the peptides influence a woman's moods. Besides being the cause of an abnormal estrogen/progesterone balance in the last half of the menstrual cycle, the brain's neuroendocrine mechanisms may also be responsible for irregular menstrual flows (oligomenorrhea) or complete loss of menstruation (amenorrhea).

These remarkable insights from Drs. Reid and Yen were made possible by the availability of new information about the brain, pituitary, and ovarian hormones, and by the existence of modern technological testing methods that enable researchers to measure minute hormonal levels in the body.

# Conditions That Influence PMS

A woman's lifestyle, her particular biology, and events in her medical history all contribute to the intensity of her premenstrual syndrome, if she is a sufferer. While she may not be directly able to control the hormonal flows within her body, a woman may have some secondary power over her biochemistry. By understanding that PMS reacts to certain influences, a

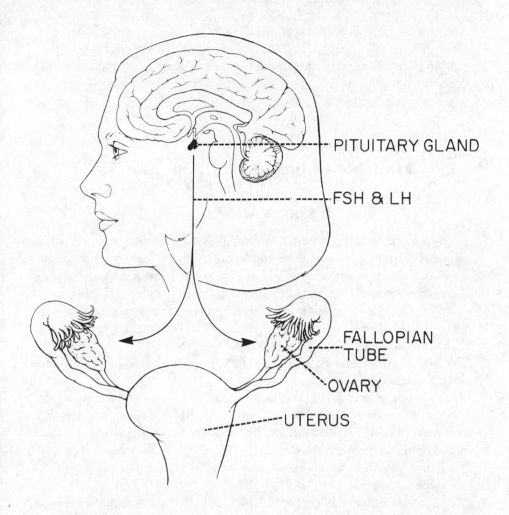

PITUITARY GLAND

FSH & LH

FALLOPIAN TUBE

OVARY

UTERUS

*How Brain Hormones Influence the Menstrual Cycle:* There is a close interaction between the brain hormones and the reproductive organs that control menstruation. There are releasing hormones in the brain that control the secretion of FSH and LH from the pituitary gland. These hormones will stimulate the ovaries to produce estrogen and progesterone, which, in turn, will stimulate the uterus to build up the endometrium (the uterine lining). It is the endometrium that is expelled as menstrual blood. If a woman is under stress, the FSH and LH will not be released and menstruation will not occur. This absence of menstruation does not mean that blood is building up inside a woman. No menstrual blood is produced when the brain hormones are blocked. There is such a close interaction between the brain and the menstrual pattern that a group of women living together and sharing similar experiences in a college dormitory might find that their menstrual cycles are synchronized. (Reproduced from *Listen to Your Body,* Fireside/Simon & Schuster, Inc., 1982.)

woman may gain insights into which of these variables she can change or alter to alleviate her symptoms. These influences also clearly indicate how premenstrual syndrome is so undoubtedly a mind/body condition, one that encompasses physical and psychological symptoms that are finally being recognized by science.

# How Your Lifestyle Influences PMS

## STRESS AND PMS

The hypothalamus in the brain masterminds the menstrual cycle. It is the hypothalamus that stimulates the secretion of the Releasing Factor, now believed to be a gonadotropin, GnRH, which in turn triggers the release of the brain hormones FSH and LH from the pituitary, and the cycle thereby is set in motion. However, any form of stress can affect the sensitive hypothalamus. Also, according to the Reid/Yen theory described in "The Power of the Brain" section of this chapter, peptides in the brain are influenced by stress before they send nerve-transmitting signals that affect the interaction of the hypothalamus and the pituitary.

Considering that the brain signals that regulate hormonal fluctuations are susceptible to stress factors at the start, and that PMS springs from the resulting hormonal fluctuations, *without a doubt* stress aggravates the syndrome. Stress inhibits the release of hormones and an inadequate supply of hormones can lead to the kind of hormonal imbalance that worsens PMS symptoms.

A woman's hormonal levels may switch from normal to slightly askew to severely imbalanced if she is thrust into particularly stress-provoking situations, or if her personal environment is stressful. Women who suffer with PMS are often under constant pressure at work, or having family problems, or they are facing major life changes such as separation, a move, divorce, and sometimes death of a loved one.

It is important for a woman to try to understand her symptoms, de-stress herself, and begin a recovery. She must attempt to change the stress-provoking elements in her life in order to unblock the brain hormones that are preventing her ovaries from producing the needed estrogen and progesterone. Some women might benefit from vitamin supplements, which have been known to work as calming agents. Patients have been helped by vitamin E, 800 to 1,000 units a day; vitamin D, 400 units a day; calcium, 2 to 3 grams a day; vitamin B-complex with extra vitamin $B_6$, 300 to 800 milligrams a day; and possibly zinc, 50 milligrams a day, and vitamin C, 1,000 milligrams a day.

By taking extra vitamins and enrolling in exercise and relaxation programs such as stretching or yoga classes, a woman may transform the way her body feels and reverse the course of her PMS. (Other methods of stress reduction are explored in Chapter 5.)

## PHYSICAL FITNESS AND PMS

It is generally believed that if a woman is in good physical condition, she will rarely experience premenstrual syndrome or she will only notice mild symptoms. Doctors always encourage women to schedule exercise programs into their daily routines. However, while it is true that physically fit women usually have few complaints about premenstrual problems, sometimes women who appear to be in excellent shape say that they exercise and still suffer from PMS. The question is: How much does a woman exercise? Physical exertion can be overdone to the point of causing hormonal imbalance.

When excessive physical activity, such as jogging, cycling, strenuous dance, results in complete amenorrhea, the disappearance of menstruation, periods probably stop because the constant exercise causes weight loss and a change in hormone balance. This hormonal shift blocks the release of the brain hormones FSH and LH. Women who are physically active need high blood counts to carry added oxygen to their muscles, and a woman who is not menstruating usually has a blood count that is higher than average. So, nature is adjusting to bodily need. The body is also protecting itself by providing less chance for anemia (a low blood count) to occur. If a thin, active woman menstruates and experiences a heavy loss of blood, she may easily become anemic.

Also, the hormonal change that causes amenorrhea may influence premenstrual syndrome. Although a woman with amenorrhea is less likely to experience PMS, she is not immune to the syndrome. Her body is building up estrogen, which is remaining in her system because she does not have a monthly menstrual flow. If she becomes tense and headachy, she is showing signs of PMS from an estrogen overload, and a reduction of physical activity may make an important difference.

Moderation in exercise is one way to keep PMS in check. Hormones, especially those in the brain, are extremely sensitive to a woman's daily regimens—diet, exercise, sleep patterns—and these hormones can rise or fall if a woman suddenly allows a routine activity either to become excessive or to vanish. Some exercise can enhance the menstrual cycle by alleviating the stress that might disrupt the body's hormonal balance, but if a woman notices that her inner harmony or her menstrual flow become radically different, she should think about whether her chosen exercise program should be modified.

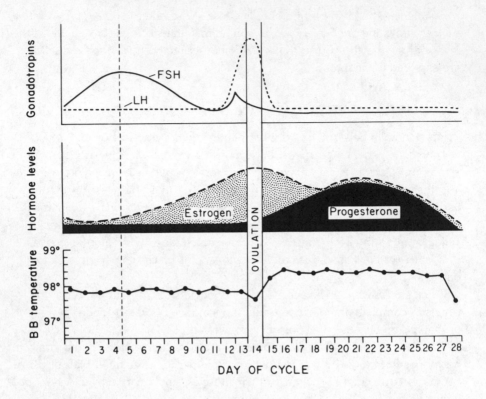

*Hormone Fluctuation During the Menstrual Cycle:* The top curves illustrate the fluctuations in the gonadotropins, the brain hormones, during the menstrual cycle. The middle curves indicate the fluctuations of the female hormones—estrogen and progesterone—during the 28-day cycle. The bottom curve indicates the basal body temperature (BBT) fluctuation. Day 1 marks the first day of menstrual bleeding. The FSH will stimulate estrogen production from the ovaries. The estrogen, in turn, will prime the cervix and increase the cervical mucus in preparation for ovulation. When the estrogen reaches a peak, it will trigger LH release. The LH will then stimulate ovulation. After ovulation, the estrogen and progesterone will increase and cause the body temperature to rise, a sign that ovulation has taken place. (Reproduced from *Listen to Your Body,* Fireside/Simon & Schuster, Inc., 1982.)

A study of 748 female students at Helsinki University in Finland shows that women who participate in sports such as hiking, cross-country skiing, and swimming tremendously increase the circulation of their blood and the oxygenating capacity of their lungs. The brain, when supplied with newly oxygenated blood, is able to cope with events that might otherwise be considered stressful enough to create a hormonal imbalance. The researchers found that symptoms of central nervous system tension lessened for women in sports, whereas the women who participated in gymnastics displayed fairly unchanging tension levels. Gymnastics, which took less time than the other, more strenuous sports in the study, benefited skeletal muscles more than the brain. The brain hormones were much more positively affected by the sports. Sportswomen who complained of headaches found relief after their workouts.

Noting this study, women who feel that their PMS complaints center around tension, irritability, and headaches might investigate the availability of sports programs in their areas. However, it really does not matter which activity she chooses, as long as a woman physically exerts herself. Moderate exercise every other day will certainly help to keep a woman's body in balance.

• **PMS and the Overweight Woman.** A woman may gain weight for many reasons. However, most of the time a woman is overweight because she overeats, not because her metabolism is changing. Eating is often her way of trying to deal with an emotional problem or a specific trouble. Food is comforting because it offers immediate, oral gratification. In our society, food is present during joyful celebrations as well as during times of mourning. It is no wonder that a woman may turn to food when she is discontented, but it is unfortunate that the foods she chooses are often nonnutritional junk foods that add on pounds. In fact, sometimes a woman who does not even binge is heavy, because the eating habits she acquired as a child gave her attachments to carbohydrates and sugary treats. And there are other weight-gaining situations.

After childbirth, or as she grows older, a woman may encounter difficulty losing weight, or a previously athletic woman may have stopped exercising and her muscle may have turned to fat. A woman with PMS may succumb to syndrome-induced food cravings that cause her to overeat and temporarily gain weight. Then there is the woman who was initially heavy—her accumulated weight may create a hormonal imbalance that contributes to premenstrual syndrome, produces more food cravings, and more weight gain. Whatever her circumstance, once a woman becomes overweight, the extra fat in her body will convert into estrogen, the female hormone.

This is what happens: The fatty tissue in an overweight woman's body enhances production of estrogen through the conversion of a biologically inactive male hormone called androstenedione, which is available in high concentration in overweight women. Androstenedione is known as an *estrogen precursor* because it is a hormone from which estrogen may be derived. This androstenedione is converted, in body fat, into *endogenous estrogen*, which is estrogen manufactured from the body tissue rather than estrogen produced by the ovaries. Another estrogen precursor, *estrone*, which is in cholesterol, activates the conversion of androstenedione, a derivative of cholesterol, into estrogen. In other words, cholesterol, which is in high concentration in fatty tissue, provides a great store of estrone, which, in turn, affects the androstenedione. The result is that a constant supply of estrogen from the fatty tissue augments the estrogen being produced by the ovaries and, to a lesser degree, by the adrenals.

With high levels of estrogen in her body, an overweight woman will clearly have an imbalance—too much estrogen and too little progesterone. She will probably experience fluid retention, swelling of the brain, and weight gain, the well-known PMS symptoms associated with an excess of estrogen.

It is therefore important for an overweight woman who is suffering from PMS to realize that if she diets and exercises, she will get rid of the fatty tissue that is contributing to her hormonal imbalance. In this way, she will be combatting her PMS while confronting her weight problem. As explained in Chapter 5, a combination of diet, exercise, and vitamins helps to fight PMS in all women, but an overweight woman might think of her PMS therapy as two things—a cure for a hormonally based condition, and a method of long-term weight reduction that is likely to be more effective than fad diets.

## Biological Influences

### AGE AND PMS

Some women have PMS symptoms in their teens, but they do not realize that they are sufferers because they have no basis of comparison. Menstruation is a new event in their lives and anything that happens may appear to be "normal." Also, PMS seems to run in families, so a mother who does not know that she is a sufferer may not be concerned if her teenage daughter behaves as she herself always has. The majority of PMS sufferers, however, are not teenagers.

Premenstrual syndrome is much more prevalent among women in their thirties than in any other age group. Women may become sufferers at any age, but usually the condition is rare among teenagers, more noticeable during the twenties, and not only common but severe in the thirties. (When women suffer from PMS during their forties, they frequently mistake the condition for menopause. See Chapter 4.)

As mentioned in the "PMS and the Overweight Woman" section, fatty tissue contributes to an increase of estrogen in the body, so as a woman gets older and slowly gains weight, she may suddenly experience symptoms caused by an overproduction of estrogen and she may realize that she did not notice these symptoms when she was younger and slimmer. Age changes the body in many ways. As a woman matures, her ovulation might not be as perfect as it was in her youth. A woman's ovaries do not function in the same way from month to month, and certainly not from decade to decade. An over-thirty woman may experience a hormonal imbalance because she is producing less progesterone than she used to. The lowered progesterone in relation to the combined ovarian and "body fat" estrogen becomes a much less effective hormone and an estrogen/progesterone imbalance occurs that contributes to premenstrual syndrome.

Then there is another reason why a woman may experience PMS for the first time when she is over thirty. Besides the fact that her ovaries are aging, and even if she has not gained weight, she may develop premenstrual syndrome because the ratio of muscle to fat in her body has changed. When a woman is young, muscle surpasses fat, but as she matures, the ratio reverses and she has more fat than muscle. (Sometimes this ratio reversal means that she gains weight too.) Once again, the passage of time is responsible.

Also, early in life a woman has her childbearing ahead of her. Older women who have borne more than one child may find that they have PMS symptoms that can be traced back to their pregnancies. Abdominal bloating is especially noticed among women who have given birth to more than one child, because pelvic congestion tends to afflict these women. In addition, it is common to see premenstrual syndrome occurring after a woman has had her normal hormonal cycle interrupted for some reason—pregnancy, or perhaps a few years on the birth control pill. The interruption of a woman's cycle takes time, so she is older when she notices the effects of an intrusion.

Women who become attuned to their bodies and know that premenstrual syndrome might surface when they are over thirty feel ready to overcome their symptoms. Before the fact that PMS might appear for the first time in an over-thirty woman was recognized, doctors prescribed tranquilizers for complaining older women and made them feel as if they might possibly be going mad. Today both doctors and patients know that PMS is more likely to strike the mother of a teenage daughter, rather than the teenage daughter herself.

## FOOD CRAVINGS AND PMS

Sometimes a woman who would never think of nibbling between meals finds herself, just before her period, munching salty potato chips, or wolfing down sugar doughnuts, or uncontrollably eating chocolate candy bars. Women with PMS are often abruptly overtaken by cravings for salt or carbohydrates, both sugars and starches, and it is not uncommon to hear sufferers say that they are "obsessed" with a desire for chocolate. As PMS sufferers know, though, succumbing to such cravings can frequently make syndromes worse.

As yet, there is no scientifically recognized reason—or reasons—for these cravings, although theories, which are described in this section, do exist. The medical profession has not officially elevated any of the current theories to the status of "fact," but many doctors, having faith in the scientific evidence that has been presented, try to give their patients what they feel are the soundest of the evaluations. A burgeoning number of doctors are trying to provide patients like Eleanor, the woman mentioned in the beginning of this chapter, with answers to the question "Why?"

• **Yearning for Salt.** It is known that the female hormone estrogen binds salt, so a woman who has premenstrual syndrome with a salt craving as one of her symptoms possibly has an overabundance of estrogen. A vicious cycle begins because estrogen causes her body to store salt, and possibly crave salt, but salt retains body fluids. A woman will start to notice that her body is becoming bloated. She may see her abdomen, hands, and feet swell from fluid retention due to salt that is being stockpiled by the estrogen. She may want to alleviate her bloatedness, but at the same time, she may feel a need to salt her foods more than usual, and to eat salted snacks. She may not realize that by consuming water-retaining salt she is increasing her body's *edema,* the medical term for fluid retention. As the body's tissues become filled with fluid, they expand and a woman gains weight. However, the more serious effects of giving in to a salt craving are migrainelike headaches and tension.

A woman can see her hands and feet swelling, but her brain, which she cannot see, is swelling too. The brain's expansion is limited by the skull that contains it, so the brain pushes out and pushes out until finally it cannot swell anymore. It stretches the surrounding brain membrane, which cannot expand beyond the skull, and it painfully irritates the membrane's sensitive nerves. Eventually, the swollen brain and stretched membrane cause a woman to have migrainelike headaches, dizziness, sensitivity to light, agitation, and a general tenseness. She may fidget and become frustrated with everyone and everything around her. In review, as the scientific studies presented in Chapter 2 show, a hormone imbalance, probably an excess of estrogen, creates an oversupply of salt, which in turn causes fluid retention that brings on serious symptoms of PMS.

A woman who has what are considered to be estrogen-induced symptoms—the bloating, weight gain from fluid retention, headaches, and tension—must realize that her salt intake has a direct relationship to the severity of her condition. By resisting the urge to eat salt, by lessening her salt consumption, she will be reducing her symptoms. There will be less salt to retain fluid and swell her body.

At the same time that a woman fights her salt craving, she should remember to drink fluids. Fluids help to cleanse the body by flushing out waste products, and if the salt level is under control, there will be little way for the consumed fluids to be retained. The equation is simple: Less salt equals less fluid retention equals less PMS. (See Chapter 5 for further information about salt and PMS.)

• ***Craving Sweets and Starches.*** When a woman surrenders to a craving for carbohydrates, especially sugary sweets, she is taking the chance of overindulging and getting symptoms of PMS that are just like symptoms of hypoglycemia. Approximately twenty to sixty minutes after she eats large amounts of refined carbohydrates and sugar, she may experience hypoglycemiclike fainting spells, fatigue, palpitation, and headaches.

According to Dr. Guy E. Abraham, in the last half of the menstrual cycle cells bind insulin. A high insulin level makes the body's blood sugar drop rapidly. A woman does not increase her blood sugar level by eating large quantities of sweets; instead, she increases her insulin. Sugar stimulates insulin production and then insulin makes the blood sugar level drop. Remember, the consumption of sugar does not raise the level of blood sugar. Refined sugar contributes to lowering blood sugar and bringing on the depression, agitation, fatigue, irritability, and headaches that are exactly like hypoglycemic episodes.

A woman may avoid these hypoglycemiclike attacks during the premenstruum, because there is a way to stop her cravings before they start. When a woman who is prone to cravings allows more than three or four hours to lapse without eating anything, she is actually giving her blood sugar time to fall and create the craving itself. However, by taking small amounts of food at approximately three-hour intervals, she will be preventing her blood sugar from dropping to the point where she feels as if she *has to have* a Snickers or a Mars bar. As just mentioned, refined sugar causes a rush of insulin, which then makes the blood sugar quickly fall. Other kinds of foods—proteins, whole grains, and carbohydrates found in vegetables—take time to metabolize into glucose, so insulin production occurs at a slow, even pace, and the blood sugar level remains steady.

Eggs, fish, poultry, and meats are high-protein foods, so by snacking on hard-boiled eggs, low-sodium tuna or chicken; or eating a slice of whole-grain bread; or selecting carbohydrate-containing vegetables such as corn, beans, potatoes, and carrots whenever possible, a woman will actually be outsmarting her endocrine system. She will not be providing her body with the "sugar fix" that brings on a surge of insulin and a rapid decline of blood sugar.

However, if a woman forgets to eat the right foods at regular intervals and she is faced with, for example, a chocolate craving, she must remember not to overdo her response to this biological call. (Even a woman who remembers to watch her diet carefully might still occasionally experience a craving.) A few bites of a Hershey bar may be enough to satisfy the body's need, although a woman may be tempted to eat an entire box of assorted chocolates.

There are also other ways to calm a craving without eating a calorie-laden food at all. Often a craving for a certain food is really the body making known its need for a specific mineral or organic chemical in which it is deficient. Since chocolate is rich in magnesium, a chocolate craving is usually a sign that the body requires this mineral, and the craving may be stilled by combination calcium/magnesium tablets. The biological reason for every craving is not known, but as reasons are discovered, doctors may be able to substitute capsules and tablets for craved foods.

There has been some belief in medical circles that a woman who craves a sweet or starchy carbohydrate may avoid pasta and take tryptophan, an amino acid that makes up serotonin, a neurotransmitter of the brain that affects mood swings. However, noted scientists have refuted this belief. Dr. Judith J. Wurtman, research scientist in the department of nutrition and food science at the Massachusetts Institute of Technology, and author of *The Carbohydrate Craver's Diet,** has been involved in the MIT research into the brain chemistry of carbohydrate hunger. According to Dr. Wurtman, when MIT volunteers who took tryptophan or an inert placebo were psychologically tested, they showed no tryptophan-induced changes in mood. Dr. Wurtman and other scientists have been conducting this research for more than a decade, and in her book she reports that it was the MIT researchers who discovered that the brain chemical serotonin, which is a mood regulator, comes from tryptophan. When a woman has a carbohydrate craving, it may be triggered by the brain's need for serotonin, but to manufacture serotonin, the brain requires tryptophan. However, tryptophan does not easily reach the brain without the aid of insulin.

Here's the process: A woman experiences a craving for sweet or starchy foods, in other words, carbohydrates. She may want cake, but if she chooses to eat a natural carbohydrate like a fruit or a vegetable, insulin will still enter her bloodstream and cause amino acids that are in the blood to depart, to leave the blood for muscles and other cells. What happens then, as Dr. Wurtman explains in her book, is that tryptophan "is one amino acid that is not affected as much by insulin secretion. Tryptophan remains in the blood after the competition has disappeared. And with the competing amino acids out of the way, the tryptophan enters the brain easily, increases the amount of

*Judith J. Wurtman, *The Carbohydrate Craver's Diet* (Boston: Houghton Mifflin, 1983).

serotonin in the brain, and the serotonin sends out a signal that shuts off the carbohydrate hunger."* Carbohydrates must be eaten alone, however, because if they are combined with protein foods, the other, abundant amino acids in protein will block the tryptophan's journey to the brain. When carbohydrates are consumed and serotonin is released, a woman will feel relaxed and calm. Serotonin is really a natural tranquilizer.

Besides the brain's hormones and neurotransmitters, another instigator of food cravings may be progesterone, the female hormone that is released in the second half of the menstrual cycle. Progesterone may change a woman's sugar tolerance so that her blood sugar level does not have far to fall before she feels a craving. Progesterone is high during pregnancy, when women are known to have extraordinary food cravings, and just before menstruation, when women are also experiencing a progesterone increase.

• **Hysteroid Dysphoria.** In December 1979, a paper entitled "Hysteroid Dysphoria," by Dr. Michael R. Liebowitz, associate professor of clinical psychiatry, and Dr. Donald F. Klein, professor of psychiatry, both with the College of Physicians and Surgeons at Columbia University in New York, appeared in the medical journal *Psychiatric Clinics of North America.* Dr. Klein identifies hysteroid dysphoria as a personality disorder that "usually but not exclusively" afflicts women. As the two doctors explain: "The hallmark of the disorder is an extreme intolerance of personal rejection, with a particular vulnerability to loss of romantic attachment." The physicians go on to report that: "When feeling rejected, these individuals experience an acute depressive, painful, crash-like reaction, characterized by loss of self-esteem and feeling extremely sad, blue, hopeless, and low. This state is accompanied by one or more of the following: overeating or craving for sweets, increased sleep or time spent in bed, a sense of leaden paralysis and inertia . . . Depressive reactions are usually short-lived (less than a week), but very frequent and repetitious, leading to severe life disruptions."

The doctors, both psychiatrists, never mention premenstrual syndrome in their study, even though they only observe women, and in spite of the fact that the symptoms of what they call hysteroid dysphoria disappear and reappear with regularity. It is remarkable that they never make the connection between the condition they have named and PMS. They even cite the fluctuation of *phenylethylamine,* one of the brain's neurotransmitters, as a possible cause of hysteroid dysphoria. Phenylethylamine, which is concentrated in chocolate, has also been identified as a possible source of PMS symptoms, but the doctors obviously prefer to believe that women suffer

*Ibid., p. 5.

"hysteroid dysphoria." Like Dickens's Miss Haversham, women are psychologically defeated because men reject them as lovers or mates, at least according to Drs. Liebowitz and Klein.

Yet of the five women who were study subjects for six months, the two who received continuous phenelzine—a drug which prevents the breakdown of phenylethylamine through the inhibition of monoamine oxidase—became the most emotionally stable and showed continued improvement of their symptoms. Phenylethylamine and amphetamine have very similar chemical structures. The doctors reported that "when depressed, hysteroid dysphorics often binge on chocolate, which is loaded with phenylethylamine." The object is to keep phenylethylamine at just the right level, because too little might cause symptoms of depression, but too much might act like amphetamine, which can at first create a "high" but after consistent use may produce a psychological state similar to paranoid schizophrenia.

If hysteroid dysphoria and premenstrual syndrome indeed turn out to be the same disease, one cannot help wondering if the drug phenelzine could be researched for use in treating women with certain PMS symptoms.

## VITAMIN DEFICIENCY AND PMS

Since the B vitamins are found mostly in liver, yeast, wheat germ, and rice polish, many American women are vitamin B deficient. The "normal" American diet is not high in organ meats, and the process of refining flour and mass-producing breads and bakery products eliminates the B vitamins. Most of the B vitamins and many other nutrients are lost in the milling or polishing process that produces white rice. (Brown rice retains the Bs.) Even as far back as the early forties, the vitamin B deficiency in the American diet was noted in medical literature. And with insufficient B vitamins, researchers discovered that the body was not effective in regulating estrogen production. Then a vicious cycle ensued because excess estrogen escalated the vitamin B deficiency, and more estrogen was produced. A resulting hormonal imbalance brought on symptoms of PMS.

Doctors could have been advising PMS patients to take vitamin B-complex for the last forty years, but there was always some skepticism as to how effective vitamins really were. Still, studies have shown that some women who suffer from PMS do find relief with vitamin B-complex, especially if they accompany it with high doses of vitamin $B_6$ (also called *pyridoxine* or *pyridoxine hydrochloride*).

The depressive symptoms that are associated with PMS, the fatigue and general malaise, have been shown to improve when a woman takes vitamin $B_6$. This vitamin disappears in cooking and canning and when foods such as whole-grain breads or cereals are stored for a long time or exposed to light. So, considering our modern food habits, it is no wonder that a woman often does not have enough $B_6$ in her body. And if for one reason or another she also has a hormonal imbalance, that imbalance may be increasing her already-existing need for vitamin $B_6$.

Pregnant women who are experiencing high progesterone levels sometimes have $B_6$ deficiencies, which make them more susceptible to morning sickness. Women who are on birth control pills with high estrogen and progesterone contents have complained of headaches, dizziness, fatigue, irritability, and depression, which are often alleviated by vitamin $B_6$. The vitamin has also been used to enhance fertility, but most recently it has been said to affect PMS in the way it influences the release of the brain's neurotransmitters, dopamine and serotonin.

The neurotransmitters are a person's mood regulators. When a woman with PMS feels irrationally tense, depressed, irritable, or agitated, she may have a vitamin $B_6$ deficiency that is decreasing the production of dopamine and serotonin. Her moods may become more stabilized after she takes this vitamin. She may even find that her food cravings and water retention subside.

Vitamin $B_6$ must be taken in high doses in combination with vitamin B-complex and other vitamins. (See Chapter 5 for vitamins and PMS.) If vitamin $B_6$ is taken alone, it might disturb the body's intestinal microorganisms and cause other B vitamins to be excreted from, rather than absorbed into, a woman's system.

There is also a possibility that a woman who has PMS might be deficient in vitamin A. In 1947, when a Dr. S. Simkins was using high doses of vitamin A as a treatment for overactive thyroid glands, he quite coincidentally discovered that his vitamin A therapy "cured" one patient's premenstrual syndrome.

Since then there have been several studies investigating the use of vitamin A in the treatment of PMS. These studies set forth different theories: that vitamin A either decreased estrogen production, or affected PMS by calming an overactive thyroid gland, or worked as a diuretic. So far, these theories have not been substantiated, because there have not been any large double-blind trials to prove that vitamin A definitely and directly affects PMS. However, that is no reason to disregard the possibility that a vitamin A deficiency may be involved in premenstrual syndrome.

## POSTPARTUM DEPRESSION AND PMS

"The first two trimesters of my pregnancy were awful, agonizing. I had morning sickness all the time," says a woman who is now undergoing treatment for premenstrual syndrome. "But my last trimester—you know, the time when most women are uncomfortable and complaining—well, I was soaring. I was enormous, bursting at the seams, but I was in seventh heaven. Then the baby came and I crashed. I had a terrible postpartum depression. It just never seemed to end."

It has been estimated that about fifty percent of the women who give birth experience what is called the *postpartum blues* at some point during the first ten days of their new motherhood. When these "blues" arrive, a woman really feels let down. She experiences fatigue, lethargy, disappointment, nervousness, and a general dissatisfaction with her life. She wants to cry and she usually loses the struggle to fight back her tears.

Most women get over their postpartum depressions in a few days, but approximately 7 to 10 percent of new mothers have very severe cases. Their depressions seem to be long-term and their symptoms appear to be very similar to the anxiety-connected PMT–A symptoms of premenstrual syndrome. And like the woman quoted above, some of the women in this extremely afflicted group may be PMS sufferers at the start, before pregnancy. A woman who lives through a practically euphoric last trimester, followed by a deep postpartum depression, is often already a PMS sufferer. However, as Dr. Katharina Dalton has concluded from her studies, a woman who does not consider herself a victim of PMS has a 90 percent chance of developing premenstrual syndrome once she has had a postpartum depression. So, just as PMS seems to indicate postpartum troubles, the postpartum blues may be a sign of forthcoming PMS.

The causes of the postpartum blues have never been exactly known. Different women suffer different degrees of depression after childbirth, depressions which seem completely unrelated to the length and intensity of their labors. In the past, it has been said that the postpartum blues arrive because once a woman gives birth she has to relinquish her spot as the center of attention to her baby, and when her position changes, she becomes depressed. Other theories blame the blues on a combination of sudden physical changes that include fatigue after childbirth, anemia, and a shift in hormones that have been steady for nine months. Dr. Dalton feels that the postpartum blues represent "a hormonal depression occurring in those women who have difficulty in adjusting to the abrupt alterations in the levels of progesterone after nine months of raised levels."*

---

*Katharina Dalton, *The Premenstrual Syndrome and Progesterone Therapy* (London: William Heinemann Medical Books Ltd., 1977), p. 120.

My feeling is that the postpartum blues probably depend upon the way a woman's emotional state after childbirth combines with her hormonal fluctuations. However, there is no way to predict who will be sure to get postpartum blues. Women who have good pregnancies and supportive families and mates usually seem to avoid postpartum depressions, but even these happy, stable, and emotionally secure women may wake up in tears one day during new motherhood and think that they have miserable lives.

Often, awareness helps women deal with the onset of postpartum depression. Women who realize that they are suffering the well-known after-childbirth blues have felt better when they have modified their diets and exercised. Since the symptoms of postpartum blues are akin to the symptoms of premenstrual syndrome, they usually respond to similar treatments.

The fact is, however, that although no one can say definitely why, women who have postpartum depressions often become PMS sufferers. Both conditions are probably due to hormonal imbalance. Certainly the awareness, exercise, and diet consciousness that help women during the postpartum blues are also beneficial during premenstrual syndrome. But in PMS cases that are extremely severe, women have reportedly responded best to progesterone treatments. The female hormone progesterone, which is high and steady during pregnancy, probably is one reason why a woman might feel so good at the end of her nine months, just before her postpartum crash. There are times when progesterone seems to emotionally return women to those pleasant, pre-childbirth days.

## STEIN-LEVENTHAL SYNDROME AND PMS

A woman who has hair on her chin and around her nipples, and pubic hairs that grow, in a triangular fashion, upward toward her navel, could be suffering from Stein-Leventhal syndrome. This condition was pinpointed by two Chicago-based physicians who diagnosed women with excessive hair growth, irregular periods, and enlarged polycystic ovaries as sufferers of the disease.

Polycystic ovaries, or *polycystic ovarian disease,* is usually a hereditary condition that often can be part of the Stein-Leventhal syndrome. The ovaries become slightly enlarged and their surfaces develop hard shells. During a normal ovulation, an egg bursts from an ovary and enters a Fallopian tube. When a woman has polycystic ovarian disease, the hard outer shell surrounding her ovary imprisons the egg and a normal ovulation cannot occur. The egg can't get out—it becomes a fluid-filled sac, a cyst inside the ovary. As more and more eggs are locked within the ovaries, more and more cysts develop and the ovaries become larger and larger. It is often difficult for a woman with polycystic ovarian disease to become pregnant, because she has an irregular ovulation pattern. About 10 to 15 percent of all women have polycystic ovarian disease. They live with irregular periods and they have exceptionally high amounts of estrogen produced by their larger ovaries.

Every woman produces estrogen, progesterone, and testosterone, and if her ovaries enlarge, they will generate more of each hormone. Sometimes, when hormonal balance is off, there is a high amount of male hormone, testosterone, secreted. The increased male hormone can cause the extra hairiness mentioned before, which signals Stein-Leventhal syndrome. A woman with this syndrome will also have irregular bleeding, and she might be overweight due to her increased hormonal production.

The hormonal imbalance of Stein-Leventhal syndrome may also bring on symptoms of premenstrual syndrome. As explained in the "PMS and the Overweight Woman" section of this chapter, fatty tissue ultimately increases estrogen. A woman with Stein-Leventhal syndrome already has a high estrogen level and a greater tendency toward breast cancer, but added weight resulting from the syndrome further increases the estrogen level in her body. Thus a woman with Stein-Leventhal syndrome has a hormonal imbalance accompanied by high salt content, fluid retention, and a greater tendency toward premenstrual syndrome.

If you have Stein-Leventhal syndrome, be alert to symptoms of PMS. Should you feel yourself suffering from PMS, try to understand the syndrome's symptoms and make an effort to combat them with a natural approach. First, attempt to keep your weight down by eating low-calorie foods and exercising, because an optimum body weight helps to counter a hormonal imbalance. If you treat yourself to a healthy diet, vitamins, and exercise but your symptoms continue to be debilitating and persistent, then you might consult a doctor you trust to find out if he thinks you need hormonal therapy.

## THE ALDOSTERONE SYSTEM AND PMS

New studies have linked PMS to an oversupply of renin, angiotensin, and aldosterone—adrenal hormones that are collectively called the *aldosterone system*. Estrogen increases the level of adrenal hormones present in the bloodstream, and an estrogen-induced aldosterone surge prevents the normal excretion of salt from the kidneys. This salt buildup then leads to fluid retention. Progesterone, on the other hand, reduces renin, angiotensin, and aldosterone and thereby activates salt excretion. In this instance, progesterone acts like a diuretic. A woman's body is carefully synchronized. If estrogen and progesterone are in perfect balance, she will experience less water retention, and possibly, less PMS.

Women with PMS are occasionally found to have high aldosterone levels in their urine, but the aldosterone levels in their blood are not significantly different from those of women without PMS. It has been theorized that the high level of urinary aldosterone may be linked to the fluctuation of the female hormones estrogen and progesterone, or may be the result of stress, since anxiety affects aldosterone excretion. This latter fact about stress brings us back to the power of the brain.

Scientists are trying to understand and control the action of dopamine, a brain chemical that reacts to stress, and indeed, may influence the flow of adrenal hormones. Studies have been done to investigate whether the drug bromocriptine, which inhibits dopamine, might lower aldosterone levels. Some of the research has shown bromocriptine to have an effect on the aldosterone system, but the drug is mainly considered for use in inhibiting the brain hormone prolactin.

New research shows that relief may come from a new drug called *spirono-lactone,* which seems to be able to counterbalance the effect of the increase in the adrenal hormones. In a study conducted at The Johns Hopkins University School of Medicine by Dr. Nelson H. Hendler, six out of seven women with PMS were freed from this condition when they used spironolactone for three months. Certainly this drug cannot be recommended in the treatment of PMS until further studies are done. The preliminary research looks promising, but one should never base a judgment on a single study.

## PROLACTIN AND PMS

Since the early seventies, scientists have thought that the brain hormone prolactin might affect premenstrual syndrome, and for years they have been trying to uncover a connection between the hormone and the condition. They discovered that prolactin fluctuates from day to day but consistently peaks when a woman ovulates and remains higher in the second half of her menstrual cycle than in the first half.

Since there was some belief that prolactin might be responsible for fluid retention, studies were done to determine whether edema could be reduced when prolactin was suppressed by the drug bromocriptine. Results have been very confusing since bromocriptine was found to be effective in some cases, ineffective in others, and occasionally even detrimental. Due to these conflict-ing results, some researchers have suggested that prolactin may play more of a part in psychological symptoms, in the depression and mood swings of PMS, than in fluid retention.

In my own practice, I have found that prolactin occasionally contributes to PMS symptoms. The serum prolactin level should always be obtained at the time a doctor requests results on the battery of hormonal blood tests that make up a routine PMS investigation. If a patient with PMS has high prolactin levels, treatment with bromocriptine should be started either daily or in a cyclic fashion when PMS symptoms appear.

## CATECHOLAMINES AND PMS

Catecholamines make up the adrenal hormones norepinephrine and epinephrine, and the brain chemical dopamine. The powerful catecholamines can affect the activity of the body's nervous system, cardiovascular system, and kidney function. Since their effects are wide-ranging, catecholamines have been researched for the ways in which they might generate the salt increase and fluid retention that accompany PMS.

Recent studies on catecholamines show that scientists are investigating every possible angle in their search for the causes of premenstrual syndrome, but in the end, the studies are complicated and inconclusive. Scientists are understanding, though, that not all symptoms of PMS can be related to fluid retention. Headache, abdominal bloating, and breast tenderness, for example, may result from specific, localized biological processes and not from systemic sources like catecholamines.

The catecholamines, which influence the involuntary nervous system, are not under a woman's control. She can do very little to increase or decrease them, although they do release during stress and shock. Adrenalin, which is closely related to epinephrine, will increase during nervousness, speed up the heart rate, and prepare the body to meet a challenge. However, it is not believed that the catecholamines, although they are involved in this process, have any significance in the development of PMS.

# Medical Influences

## THE PILL AND PMS

Years ago it was widely believed that the birth control pill was a good way to treat premenstrual syndrome, but today it appears that past studies had confused the symptoms of PMS with menstrual cramps, dysmenorrhea. The early birth control pills, which were high in estrogen, had many severe side effects, but like the modern pills, they often helped to relieve menstrual cramps. On the other hand, women with PMS frequently found that their problems either remained the same or grew worse on the pill. It has been estimated that, even now, 25 to 44 percent of the women who decide to take the pill have to change during the first year to another form of contraception, or try different types of pills, because they have so many undesirable side effects. The pill seems to either increase premenstrual syndrome or make women with tendencies toward PMS unable to tolerate the pill.

There have been two double-blind studies in which two groups of women with premenstrual problems—one on placebos and one on birth control pills—were observed. Both the women on the placebos and the women on the pill reported less premenstrual tension and irritability. Their psychological symptoms diminished, but both groups continued having the physical symptoms of PMS. It is interesting to note that several of the women on the pill described even more severe PMS discomfort on the pill than they had before taking oral contraceptives.

The hormonal contents in the latest birth control pills have been changed. Today there is less estrogen in relation to progesterone, or *progestogen,* the synthetic progesterone used in the manufacture of the pill. The problem with synthetic progesterone, progestogen, is that it lowers the body's natural progesterone level and intensifies an already existing estrogen/progesterone imbalance. A woman on the current pill is likely to suffer an increase in her particular PMS symptoms. She might have more headaches, mood swings, fatigue, depression, and weight gain. It is important to mention that many women do feel fine on the pill but that other women are not able to tolerate any oral contraceptives. This latter group of women, which usually includes PMS sufferers, should find other methods of birth control.

Dr. Katharina Dalton reports that in a hospital study in which forty-four women with premenstrual syndrome had taken the pill, forty had developed side effects. She also states that in a nationwide migraine survey in England, 81 percent of the women with menstrual migraines said that the pill had given them more painful headaches.

Women with PMS should be striving for hormonal balance in their bodies, and the pill promotes just the opposite, a hormonal *imbalance.* In fact, women have even found that when they stopped the pill, their PMS symptoms were especially bad each month and their bodies never really "bounced back."

## TUBAL STERILIZATION AND PMS

In my previous book, *Listen to Your Body,** I included some of the many letters I had received from women who had undergone tubal sterilizations and felt awful afterward. They were glad that they did not have to worry about becoming pregnant anymore, but they had found that they were often in pain

*Niels Lauersen, *Listen to Your Body,* (New York: Fireside/Simon & Schuster, Inc., 1982).

before their periods and they were distraught. They had migraine headaches and mood swings that changed their personal relationships.

The symptoms these women described matched certain symptoms of premenstrual syndrome, and indeed, it has been found that a percentage—some studies estimate as high as 37 percent—of women who have tubal sterilizations develop PMS and other complications following their surgeries. Researchers who have started to study the aftereffects of tubal sterilization have named the postoperative condition *post-tubal-ligation syndrome (PTLS).* Besides PMS, women who experience this syndrome after surgery may have pelvic pain, irregular menstrual bleeding, and galactorrhea, a milky discharge from the nipples.

If a physician cauterizes, removes, or damages too large a portion of the Fallopian tubes and their blood vessels, he will reduce blood flow, the ovaries might shrink, and women may bleed less during menstruation. A hormonal imbalance might result in abnormal ovulations with irregular menstrual bleeding. When ovulation is off, there can be decreased progesterone production which brings on premenstrual syndrome. Research has shown, in fact, that after tubal ligations women have high serum estradiol (estrogen) and low serum progesterone in the second half of their menstrual cycles, the same monthly hormonal imbalance that Drs. Israel and Dalton have cited as the cause of PMS. This hormonal dysfunction in the second half of the menstrual cycle, which is also called the *luteal phase,* might explain why a woman fails to conceive after her tubal ligation is reversed through microsurgery.

The hormonal imbalance can also result in ovarian cyst formations. Then, nerve irritation can lead to severe cyclic pelvic pain, which can become so intolerable that women agree to unnecessary surgery. Women have had D&Cs, additional laparoscopies, removal of their ovaries, and even hysterectomies to rid themselves of the problems of post-tubal-ligation syndrome, which include PMS.

Women who have premenstrual syndrome or irregular periods, women who have suffered postpartum depressions or discomfort while on birth control pills, and women who have family histories of PMS are very likely to have hormonal imbalances. I would discourage these women from undergoing tubal sterilizations because they are at especially high risk of becoming more severely hormonally imbalanced after surgery. I have seen too many women suffer emotionally and physically after tubal sterilizations. This is one time when a woman may be able to stop premenstrual syndrome before it starts.

## HYSTERECTOMY AND PMS

It may be that in about one-third of the hysterectomies performed, healthy uteri are removed, and it is my constant recommendation that second opinions be sought in connection with hysterectomies. Since most hysterectomies are elective, not life-or-death surgeries, there is usually a month from the moment the decision to proceed with the operation is made to the scheduled date of surgery. Although there are times when a hysterectomy is a lifesaving measure or a way to protect a woman's health, the fact that hysterectomy is the most performed *major* surgery for women is shocking. Hysterectomies are advised much too blithely. A uterus should never be removed as a means of contraception or, least of all, as a means of ending the agony of premenstrual syndrome. For one thing, it will not work. A woman will still have symptoms of PMS.

The uterus is a functioning part of the menstrual cycle. The blood supply to the ovaries comes through the uterus, and when a woman's uterus is removed, her ovaries receive less blood and they perform irregularly. They continue to produce hormones, but since a part of the finely tuned feminine system is gone, the hormones fluctuate erratically and a woman finds that she has mood swings, depression, and other problems of premenstrual syndrome. If she was a PMS sufferer before her surgery, she might even recognize a return of her symptoms in a cyclic pattern similar to her monthly menstrual cycle. Her brain hormones are still operating, even though they are no longer beautifully synchronized.

Whether or not a woman's hysterectomy included the removal of her ovaries, about a week after surgery she will have a surge of FSH, followed by a release of LH a few days later. However, with organs that used to trigger and halt hormonal flows now missing, the brain hormones go awry. Three weeks later, FSH rushes into the body three times more heavily than it usually does and LH appears in twice the amount it used to. This severe hormonal discord can make a woman think she is going crazy. She may begin to feel as if she is reliving her premenstrual days, and this feeling, which brings inner turmoil along with it, can go on for years.

If a woman undergoes a hysterectomy in which both ovaries are removed, she will be involved in a surgical "castration." She will instantly enter menopause and never again experience menstruation. Once the ovaries, which produce female hormones and eggs, are surgically excised, female hormone production stops. A woman might have felt fine before her hysterectomy, but after she might find herself overcome with hot flushes, backache, and depression. If the after-surgery symptoms include hot flushes, a woman is experiencing surgical menopause. The postsurgical PMS condition excludes the hot flushes of menopause.

Often, women who are put into surgical menopause gain weight, because they are distraught, do not feel well, and eat to overcome their emotional difficulties. Fatigue and loss of energy are also intensified after surgical menopause. Sugar provides a temporary lift, and women, because they are tired, may continue to eat. Increased body weight may then lead to high blood pressure and even heart disease if care is not taken. Due to all the grave potential problems associated with hysterectomy, a woman should make every effort to keep her reproductive system intact.

The significant psychological impact of a hysterectomy often does not show up until three months to three years after surgery. By then a woman may have experienced a reduced sex drive because, if her ovaries were removed, her hormone production stopped. Without her hormones, her sexual despondency is physically, not psychologically, rooted, but she may experience psychic despair because her sexuality has changed. During the excitement phase of sexual arousal, the uterus becomes engorged with blood much in the way a man's penis does when he is sexually stimulated. Without her uterus, a woman might feel as if her body is not as sexually responsive. Also, unless women have had cancer, they often wrestle with the question of whether or not their hysterectomy was really necessary. If a woman begins to conclude that her operation was superfluous, then she may experience rage, depression, or both. For emotional as well as physical reasons, a woman should be very cautious about agreeing to a hysterectomy.

Many different conditions and changes in a woman's body can lead to premenstrual syndrome. The syndrome may arise from a hormonal imbalance, but there are so many other influences to consider that it is hard to say whether PMS is caused by one single factor or a combination of factors.

It is hoped that this chapter may help a woman to see that the symptoms she is experiencing during her premenstruum may be connected to many diverse bodily functions, as well as to her lifestyle and her medical history. Every woman's syndrome is unique. Knowing this, a woman might try to become a partner with her doctor. Together, a woman and her doctor might share a commitment to find the cause of her PMS, and the treatment that is right for her.

# 4

---

# How to Know If You Have PMS

Women who discover that they have premenstrual syndrome never forget the moment when they realized they were sufferers. Some women were desperately worried that they were seriously ill, while others considered themselves to be moody, depressed people with a lot of "bad days." Then something happened, either they or their loved ones heard about PMS and these women began to have hope that their lives would be different.

Three such women, who asked that their real names not be used, vividly remember feeling exhilarated when they learned about PMS because they realized they were being given a chance to be well. These women, fictitiously named Nancy, Pamela, and Ann, are in the vanguard of the medical profession's recognition of PMS. Their cases are more severe than most and they are brave to speak out. Like other women who are seeking diagnoses for this controversial condition, they are forerunners in the field of women's health. Their loved ones do not think they are people who are clinging to PMS as an excuse for physical complaints and mood swings, because anyone who is close to a PMS sufferer can see healthy improvements after diagnosis and treatment. These women do not want to deny themselves the opportunity to investigate what for them might be "a way out."

Everyone must become aware of what PMS really is and how it strikes. Symptoms vary in degree from month to month and from woman to woman. Discovering that you have PMS is often the first step toward relief, but the syndrome, as Nancy, Pamela, and Ann's stories show, is not always easy to spot, since it is often mistaken for other conditions.

## WHAT THEY WENT THROUGH—REAL STORIES OF PMS SUFFERERS

• ***Nancy's Story.*** "I'm thirty-three years old and I'm just beginning to see that my symptoms probably started far back into my teens." Nancy is a divorced mother with a ten-year-old son. She works in a real estate office with three other people who know that when she is irritable and frustrated they had better "back off," she says. She never knew why she had so many bad moods, and why she was angry so often. Her co-workers adjusted themselves to her changing temperament and even Nancy's son left her alone when she was touchy. "I wanted him to stay away from me, but I couldn't tell him why," says Nancy, "because until recently I didn't know myself."

Nancy's sister Claire read about PMS in women's magazines after she had heard about the British murder trials. Nancy had always thought that Claire was impossible to live with, and when Claire decided that she probably had PMS, she gently told Nancy that their personalities were similar. Claire even thought that premenstrual syndrome ran in their family, that she, their mother, and Nancy all had it.

"I started thinking that maybe Claire was right, but I wasn't very serious about considering premenstrual syndrome a problem of mine until last month, when I went over the edge," says Nancy. "I became violent. I'm usually not so out of control. I can almost always head off trouble, but this time I didn't do it. I stabbed my boyfriend in the leg. I walked right into the kitchen, got the carving knife, and stabbed him. Then I knew I needed help."

Luckily, Nancy did not permanently injure the man. He left and even refused to get stitches, because he was embarrassed over the incident. Meanwhile, Nancy remained upset and distraught. "It was all too intense," she says. "The next day, I got my period and felt calm and happy. Then I knew Claire was correct. I was just beside myself the night before. We were having an argument over someone he wanted to invite to dinner, a woman whom I don't like. He just kept insisting that I tell him *why* I didn't want her around. I tried to go to sleep to stop the argument, but he stood at the foot of my bed and kept talking. I couldn't stand it anymore. I had to stop him or I was going to explode." That's when she stormed into the kitchen and pulled the knife from its holder.

In consultation with a doctor a week later, Nancy realized that her symptoms started two weeks before her period and grew worse as her menstruation neared. She now understands that the two or three days before she begins to flow are incredibly stressful times that exhaust her body and her mind. Every month, during the last half of her cycle she experiences a great deal of water retention that makes her puffy all over. She has a constant pressure pain down her left leg, the kind of discomfort that usually comes with pregnancy, and then she has cramps. But the physical symptoms do not concern her as much as the emotional ones, the anger.

"I don't cry and weep, I become enraged, and my fury builds as my cycle winds down," says Nancy. Since the stabbing incident, her boyfriend has forgiven her but she has not forgiven herself. "I can't believe I did that, but now I have to live with it and I have to come to terms with my actions. I'm working with my doctor, keeping a calendar of symptoms and taking vitamins. He's going to figure out my treatment after he looks at my calendar and does more testing. At least now I know what's happening. I've explained PMS to my boyfriend, my son, and my boss. They're all going to help me try to deal with it. I just can't be so out of control ever again."

• *Pamela's Story.* She had been reading about premenstrual syndrome for well over a year, but Pamela still was not completely connecting her problems with PMS. Then her mother began researching the condition, mailing articles and flyers to her, and her husband said that he saw cycles in her behavior. "He really noticed the patterns much more than I did," says Pamela.

Today she looks back and can definitely say that for at least three years she has been involved in two-week-cycle patterns. "I start having symptoms two weeks before my period, usually when I'm ovulating," says Pamela. "What was happening before I started treatment was that for two weeks after my ovulation I got a slow, gradual feeling of separating from myself. I steadily lost control over what I was doing. I'd become like two people. I wouldn't be whole, and these severe, schizophreniclike symptoms would often lead to violence."

Pamela lashed out at the people closest to her when what she now knows is her PMS overtook her. She would yell at her boyfriend, now her husband, call him names, hit him, bite him to the point of drawing blood. "I didn't mean it. I would not believe what would come out of my mouth," says Pamela. "I'd think, why did I say that? I got a very strange feeling and with that feeling came a fear that I was going to hurt somebody very badly. Psychologically, I became very timid. Afraid of my shadow. And that fear added to all my other symptoms. I was very near suicide, seriously contemplating it because to live two weeks out of every month not knowing what you're going to do is no way to live. I thought that if I couldn't correct this problem, I'd be helping people by killing myself."

Eight years ago, when she was twenty-one, Pamela was diagnosed as having hypoglycemia. The diet and vitamins for hypoglycemia helped alleviate the torturous monthly changes that doctors at the time did not connect to PMS, but the remedies did not bring permanent relief. At twenty-nine, Pamela was losing her will to live when, in desperation, she decided to see a doctor.

Besides her Jekyll-and-Hyde symptoms, Pamela also suffered breast tenderness, headaches, and bloatedness. After three months on hormonal therapy, a treatment that is discussed in Chapter 5, Pamela does not experience physical ailments or that horrible loss of self she used to feel. Like Nancy, she was urged by her loved ones to find out whether her symptoms were caused by PMS. Now Pamela feels that she needs to know more than she has already learned. "I'm like a person who has experienced some kind of seizure and then regains consciousness. Now I'm back to myself and I have questions, doubts, guilts, and confusions. Until I get some answers, until I figure out what this condition is all about, I won't be able to stop blaming myself."

• **Ann's Story.** When Ann was seventeen, she was put on the birth control pill; she went off it at age twenty. Then her troubles really began. At thirty, she can look back over ten years of misery. "I was diagnosed as having severe mental and emotional problems and I was put on antipsychotics, mood stabilizers, and tranquilizers of all kinds," says Ann. "My family and my friends were always convincing me, almost brainwashing me, that if I stayed on my medication, I would be all right. They would compare me to a diabetic who had to be on insulin. I would have to be on tranquilizers for the rest of my life. And I hate being dependent. I felt out of control of my body and now I know why. I *was* out of control. For so long."

Ann's three children, ages eight, four, and thirteen months, were her main concern. She chose to undergo psychiatric care because she was so afraid she might hurt them. "My symptoms were anxiety, depression, anger, hostility, and violent outbursts," says Ann. "I had a time when I lived in dire fear that I was going to cross that fine line between discipline and child abuse. I was verbally abusive toward my husband, but I would really thrash out at the kids. When I had these outbursts I tended to observe myself. I felt like a third party, looking at what I was doing. There was nothing I could do about it. I was not in control of my actions. It's like somebody else is taking over. You know you're lashing out at your kids, but you also know that there's not a damn way you can stop yourself."

The first time Ann heard about PMS was on a television talk show, where the guests were debating the murder trials of England. They began to describe the syndrome's symptoms and Ann became mesmerized. "The things they were discussing were so close to what I was going through, it was a little spooky," she says. At the time, she wrote down the telephone numbers of clinics where PMS was being treated but she did not investigate any further. The day she decided to look into premenstrual syndrome was the day she woke up and realized that she had not succeeded in killing herself.

"I attempted suicide because I felt that there was no hope," says Ann. "I was destroying my family and I thought that the world would be better off without me. I couldn't go on living like that anymore. The doctors and psychiatrists didn't know what to do. Nothing was working." Ann took an overdose of tranquilizers, but her husband was home at the time and he rushed her to the emergency room of a local hospital, where doctors pumped her stomach and saved her life.

After her recovery, Ann visited a PMS clinic and cried when she left. "I was crying for two reasons," she says. "One was for joy, because I could finally believe that I was not crazy. I always thought I wasn't crazy but I didn't know how to tell the world. The second reason was that I was very, very scared that the treatment would not work."

It took ten years for Ann to link her symptoms with premenstrual syndrome, but after six months of treatment she is a transformed woman. Her hormonal therapy changed her relationship with her husband and her children, but as she says, "Most important, it changed my attitude toward myself. I never thought I had what it takes to go out into the world, have a career, do things for myself—but I have that ability." How wonderful that her self-discovery did not have to wait another ten years.

## WHEN TO SUSPECT PMS

Neither Nancy, Pamela, nor Ann were quick to think that they had premenstrual syndrome. They attributed their symptoms to other causes without ever asking their gynecologists if they were possibly sufferers. Doctors also neglected to make the PMS connection, and the women continued to assume that they were psychologically damaged, emotionally impaired. Ann, who had an especially severe case of premenstrual syndrome, was given drugs that probably served to cloud her judgment while she was being "calmed down." However, over time these women became courageous enough to believe that they might have a hormonally based problem, and then they were strong and assertive in describing their symptoms. Each woman was also willing to chart her symptoms on a calendar and work hand in hand with her physician.

Diagnosis and treatment of premenstrual syndrome are not yet exact sciences and today's patients and doctors must strive for results together. A woman may have emotional and physical symptoms that vary in severity from month to month, and she must not be afraid that she will be considered "mad" if she discusses them with her doctor. Also, if she has symptom-free intervals every month, a pattern that is a definite and necessary sign of PMS, she will be even more secure in her mind that she is a sufferer.

However, while it is true that a woman who has an inkling that she might have PMS may be afflicted with one or many of the wide spectrum of symptoms that are carefully detailed in this chapter, she may also have other menstrual problems. Before she seeks help, a woman should be aware that menstrual cramps, endometriosis, and menopause are all conditions that, like premenstrual syndrome, are labeled *menstrual distress,* but they are not part of PMS.

A woman must remember that it is because the menstrual cycle exists that the conditions classified as menstrual distress exist. She might review "The Ebb and Flow of the Menstrual Cycle" in Chapter 3 to gain an understanding of how, month after month, her menstrual cycle follows the carefully planned course of nature. However, within this course there are many opportunities for things to go wrong.

The menstrual cycle is orchestrated by delicately balanced, precisely flowing hormones that may begin to climb and fall erratically. Also, organs may not function as they should. Symptoms may arise that signal menstrual cramps (dsymenorrhea), endometriosis, or the perimenopausal stage, and all of these conditions may appear without premenstrual syndrome. A woman must familiarize herself with these conditions to have a better idea of what her problem might be. She might be suffering from other types of menstrual distress and not have PMS at all, or she might have premenstrual syndrome in addition to another condition. The different forms of menstrual distress can be present alone or in combination with each other.

Since she may become confused by her symptoms, a woman might set aside time to relax and read the next two sections, "Menstrual Distress Is More Than PMS" and "Recognizing the Symptoms of PMS," which should give her insights into what might be troubling her. The next section in particular aims to separate PMS from menstrual cramps, endometriosis, and perimenopausal and menopausal symptoms, define these conditions, and end the mix-up of menstrual distress.

## MENSTRUAL DISTRESS IS MORE THAN PMS

*Menstrual distress,* as mentioned in Chapter 2, is an umbrella term used to describe many problems a woman might have in connection with her menstrual period. Premenstrual syndrome, menstrual cramps (dysmenorrhea), endometriosis, and perimenopausal or menopausal symptoms all fall under the category of menstrual distress.

The symptoms of premenstrual syndrome, which are carefully detailed in this chapter, are separate from other forms of menstrual distress. It is important for a woman to be able to differentiate among the conditions and understand how they may sometimes affect each other, in order to tell as accurately as possible whether or not she has PMS.

• **PMS vs. Menstrual Cramps.** A woman may suffer premenstrual syndrome in combination with menstrual cramps, or she may experience either condition alone. However, she should try not to confuse the two because, first of all, they spring from different sources.

Scientists recently discovered that cramp-causing, hormonelike substances called prostaglandins, which are produced in many tissues of the body, are significantly present in the lining of the uterus. Women who have excruciating menstrual cramps have been found to have more prostaglandins than women who were less bothered. PMS, on the other hand, is never mentioned in connection with prostaglandins. Premenstrual syndrome had been linked to hormonal imbalances and changes in interactions between brain hormones and the body's neuroendocrine system.

The symptoms of PMS are illustrated in the figure on page 37 and are also detailed in this chapter. Women who endure monthly attacks of cramps may sometimes have nausea, vomiting, diarrhea, headache, fatigue, and nervousness in addition. Headache, fatigue, and nervousness are occasionally observed as symptoms of premenstrual syndrome, but they are not accompanied by cramps. Also, while PMS sufferers notice symptoms anywhere from two to fourteen days before menstruation, women with menstrual cramps do not experience symptoms until their periods are about to begin.

During most of the monthly cycle, cramp-causing prostaglandins are held in check by the hormone progesterone. But just before menstruation, progesterone drops and prostaglandins rise. The cervix, the mouth of the womb from which the blood usually flows, tightens. The prostaglandins in the menstrual blood trapped within the womb are absorbed by the uterine muscles, released, reabsorbed, and released again in a circular fashion. It's a vicious cycle. As the prostaglandins follow their circuit, the uterus contracts and cramps with ever more intensity, and until the menstrual blood flows from the vagina, taking with it the prostaglandins, women feel terrible. They are suffering very real pain, which is clinically called primary dysmenorrhea. (Secondary dysmenorrhea involves pain brought on by a pelvic disorder such as infection, endometriosis, fibroid tumors pressing on nerves, or a poorly placed IUD.)

As prostaglandins are released, the uterus contracts and cramps, resulting in what might be called a charley horse of the womb. Sometimes the uterine contractions can be more pronounced than they are during childbirth. And if the blood is not allowed to escape through the vagina, it could back up, first into the Fallopian tubes and then into the abdominal cavity, making already unbearable cramps even more blindingly painful. This backup could eventually lead to endometriosis, which is explained in the next section.

Every woman who is suffering menstrual cramps or any of the accompanying symptoms should see her doctor to make sure that her abdominal pain is not being caused by infection or tumors or one of several different types of pelvic diseases. If a doctor can rule out serious pelvic problems, then prostaglandins are probably the cause and a woman can be treated.

Scientists have discovered that aspirinlike medication prevents the body from releasing prostaglandins. In fact, a woman who has not tried aspirin might take two aspirins four times a day for two days *before* her period starts, and during the first days of her flow. Prostaglandins will not be blocked unless the aspirin, or any other antiprostaglandin drug, is taken *before menstruation*. Timing is essential for treatment.

Women have also been helped by Midol, the time-honored, over-the-counter, aspirinlike menstrual-pain reliever. Doctors did not know that Midol was actually lowering the prostaglandin level for women all these years, but indeed it does. Two Midol tablets four times a day, two days *before* and during the first few days of menstruation, have been known to provide positive changes. The antispasmodic in Midol also enhances its effects. Once again, it is essential for a woman to monitor her body for the arrival of her period, because she will have a much better chance for relief if she takes antiprostaglandin medicine *prior to menstruation*.

Three prescription drugs recently approved by the FDA for dysmenorrhea—Motrin (ibuprofen), Anaprox (naproxen sodium), and Ponstel (mefenamic acid)—are often more effective than aspirin in blocking prostaglandins. One to two tablets of either drug, taken four times a day before menstruation and continued during the first few days of bleeding, should work their magic. Besides curbing cramps, these drugs also reduce menstrual flow. Since the drugs can irritate the stomach, they should be taken with some food, a cracker, or a glass of milk.

Each woman must listen to her body and decide how many tablets she needs for her own menstrual problem. She might even change her dosage from month to month. With the intense research that is currently being conducted, a variety of prescription and nonprescription antiprostaglandin medications will probably be available in the near future. For now, however, it is important to remember that Motrin, Anaprox, Ponstel, and Midol, taken properly, can act like wonder drugs. They can exorcise the menstrual pain that grips perfectly healthy women.

• **PMS vs. Endometriosis.** Endometriosis, just like menstrual cramps, may exist alone or in combination with premenstrual syndrome, or there is a third alternative—some women have endometriosis, menstrual cramps, and premenstrual syndrome together during every menstrual cycle. These women suffer terribly.

Endometriosis is a disease in which the tissue that forms the endometrium, the lining of the uterus, spreads to the organs outside the womb. As explained in Chapter 3, during the last half of a woman's menstrual cycle—the two weeks that begin with ovulation and end in menstruation—the lining of the uterus grows rich in glandular tissue and blood vessels. Steadily, naturally, an emerging vascular layer turns the endometrium into a soft, spongy nest, a bed for a fertilized egg.

At this point, the endometrium exists to nurture fertilization, so if an egg is not fertilized, the body has no reason to keep this enriched lining. The cycle comes to an end. A woman's uterus begins rhythmic contractions that disturb the blood supply to the uterine lining and cause the unused endometrium to detach from the womb and leave the body as menstrual blood.

When a woman is healthy, the regular contractions of her uterus push the uterine lining, the sloughed-off endometrium, first through the cervix, the mouth of the womb, and then through her vagina. But a woman who gets endometriosis often has a constricted uterus and a tight cervix, which do not let all the menstrual blood escape vaginally. Instead, a portion of the blood-filled uterine lining is pushed backward through the Fallopian tubes and sprayed out the tubes into the abdomen. Such a woman usually has a history of menstrual cramps.

As mentioned a moment ago, women with severe menstrual cramps have in their uterine linings high levels of prostaglandins, which can produce contractions similar to the ones experienced during labor and childbirth. In these women, the chances are great that their blindingly painful contractions will push the endometrial tissue into places where it can run wild. Endometrial tissue that has been flushed into the Fallopian tubes and sprayed out into a woman's abdomen can implant itself on her ovaries, on the outside of her uterus, and in the cavity between the uterus and the rectum called the cul-de-sac. The tissue can begin to grow like a transplant on any of its new locations, and once that happens, endometriosis has begun. It should be noted, however, that even if a woman does not have severe cramps, tissue can still be pushed backward into the abdomen to cause endometriosis.

Each month, the fluctuation of the hormones estrogen and progesterone, which causes the production of the endometrium inside the uterus, is also having an effect on the endometriosis outside the uterus. The tissue thickens, bleeds, and, since it has no escape, spreads throughout the abdominal cavity. Sometimes, as it expands and bleeds, the tissue breaks off in cystic chunks that implant themselves elsewhere and cause severe abdominal pain.

An endometrical mass spreading behind a uterus can pull and tilt the womb backward. The tissue can move into the ovaries and Fallopian tubes, where it causes infertility. Endometriosis can even enter into the bowls and create bloody stools and pain during peristalsis, bowel movement. The tissue can penetrate the wall of the bladder, grow into the bladder, and then attack the kidneys and rectum. There have also been cases where endometriosis has spread to the lungs and—unbelievable as it may seem—the brain. If left untreated for years, endometrial tissue can even become cancerous.

However, if a woman can monitor her body for the distinct symptoms of the hidden disease, as endometriosis is called, she can possibly catch it at an early and curable stage. The symptoms of the disease include a possible painful ovulation two weeks before menstruation, severe cramps during menstruation, and a deep abdominal pain on one side or the other or an unspecific abdominal pain before or after menstruation. Other signs are infertility and pain during sexual intercourse. Many women who are infertile and are told they have no physical defects may, indeed, have endometriosis. During the course of the disease, pelvic pain caused by pressure on a woman's organs and nerves slowly intensifies.

The main treatment used by knowledgeable doctors today involves a new, breakthrough drug called Danocrine (danazol), a synthetic derivative of the male hormone testosterone, which stops ovulation and gives a woman a "pelvic rest." Danazol, which is the generic name for the drug, blocks the release of the brain hormones FSH and LH, which set the menstrual cycle in motion. A woman's ovaries are not stimulated to release an egg, so there is no ovulation and estrogen and progesterone hormones do not increase. Estrogen and progesterone remain on the same steady low levels that are normally found after menstruation, a time when most women feel their best. When a woman does not ovulate and her female hormones do not fluctuate, there is no buildup of the endometrium and no chance for endometriosis to grow.

When a woman takes Danocrine—200-milligram tablets two, three, or four times daily, depending on her symptoms—for six to nine months, the endometrial tissue dies and, like all dead tissue, it is slowly reabsorbed by the body and disappears. Of course, a woman does not menstruate while she is on the medication.

Surgery should be performed as a treatment for endometriosis only when a woman has large masses that must be removed. However, a physician should not attempt extensive surgery with the goal of removing the disease totally, because he will never be able to succeed. A surgeon cannot remove every bit of endometriosis in a woman's body. After surgery, the disease will come back. A woman's doctor may tell her that he has cut, burned, or scraped all of the endometriosis away, but if a woman is not placed on danazol after her operation, the disease will always return. A woman ought to be placed on danazol therapy both before her operation, to reduce the endometrial growth, and after it, to prevent a reappearance of the disease.

It is possible that after her endometriosis has been treated a woman might develop mood swings and other symptoms of premenstrual syndrome. Fluctuation of the female hormones estrogen and progesterone affects both endometriosis and premenstrual syndrome. If a woman has—or has had—endometriosis, she may also have a hormonal imbalance and may be more prone to PMS than a woman who has never been diagnosed as someone with the hidden disease. Once a woman has endured one form of menstrual distress, she should be on the alert for signs of others, even though they are technically not related.

• *PMS vs. Menopause.* Before explaining how a woman in her forties may confuse symptoms of premenstrual syndrome with approaching menopause, it is best to define what menopause really is:

*Menopause,* which comes from the Greek *mens,* meaning monthly, and *pausa,* meaning stop, is the time when a woman's monthly menstrual period comes to a halt. When we speak about menopause, we are talking about the changes that occur in a woman after she stops menstruating.

Menopause can last anywhere from one year to several years, varying from one woman to another. It is the time when a woman may experience the well-known change-of-life symptoms such as hot flashes, hot flushes, dry skin, backaches, and other problems associated with declining estrogen levels. Some women, particularly women who have no obvious symptoms of menopause, might never know when menopause begins and ends because they are able to pass through this phase with little or only minimal discomfort.

The time prior to the complete cessation of menstruation, when a woman is noticing a change in her menstrual pattern due to the natural decline in her female hormones, is called *perimenopause*. This is a time when a woman might see irregular or so-called dysfunctional uterine bleeding. During the perimenopause, a woman might also experience mild menopausal symptoms—hot flashes, hot flushes, depression, aches and pains. The perimenopause can last anywhere from a few months to several years, although some women never experience this phase at all—one day they just stop menstruating and enter menopause.

During natural menopause, a woman should maintain a balance of calcium and phosphorus in her body. Certain foods such as cottage cheese, spinach, lobster, milk, and spaghetti contain varying quantities of these two minerals. In addition, approximately 2,600 milligrams of calcium carbonate tablets should be taken daily. Vitamin D, at least 400 units daily, will also aid in building calcium in the bones. Fluoride tablets help strengthen teeth and bones, and vitamin E—800 to 1,000 units daily—might also improve the bones. (If a woman chooses to take vitamin E, she should also add extra vitamin C to her regime since the body's supply of vitamin C is somewhat depleted by vitamin E.) Since most refined foods have been robbed of vitamin B, a vitamin B-complex containing vitamin $B_6$ would complete this supplementary regimen. Thus, a proper diet, accompanied by a regimen of supplementary calcium, fluoride, and vitamins D, B, and possibly E and C, might help to lessen the severity of menopausal symptoms. After that, exercise to strengthen the bones is essential. Bicycling and walking are good, but swimming, an activity that never strains the bones, is especially advised.

However, subtle hormonal changes occur continuously in the course of a lifetime and a woman's seeming transformations may have nothing to do with menopause. When a woman is in her forties, she may notice physical and psychological symptoms she did not experience in earlier years, but her hormonal levels may simply have changed to the point where symptoms have become apparent. It is well-known that PMS intensifies with age. Premenstrual syndrome is hardly ever seen among teenagers; the condition becomes more recognizable among women in their twenties, and it can be common as well as severe when women enter their late thirties and early forties.

Many women who experience menstrual irregularity, depression, and weight gain in their forties immediately assume that because they feel different they are in menopause. Usually these women are not premenopausal (or perimenopausal) but are suffering varying degrees of premenstrual syndrome.

Women in their forties who have gained weight, experienced major life changes, lived through stressful events, or had tubal ligations often experience the symptoms of premenstrual syndrome because weight gain, stress, and sterilization cause hormonal imbalances leading to PMS. It is important that women realize the difference between premenstrual syndrome and menopause because the two conditions require opposing treatments.

A woman with premenstrual syndrome might cut down her salt intake and take extra vitamin B-complex with $B_6$, or be prescribed progesterone supposi-tories, if they are needed. (See Chapter 5.) When it comes to hormonal therapy, there is a marked difference in the way premenstrual syndrome and menopause are treated. When a woman is suffering from PMS, her estrogen becomes too potent in relation to her progesterone and her hormonal treatment, if needed, should be progesterone. On the other hand, a woman with menopausal symptoms so severe that hormone treatment is indicated might need estrogen to curb her symptoms. Thus, if a wrong diagnosis is rendered and the wrong medication is given, a woman's condition might worsen rather than improve.

Therefore, a woman in her forties who notices menstrual irregularity should consider the possibility of premenstrual syndrome before she concludes that she is entering menopause. Although almost 10 percent of women say that the first time they notice PMS is at menopause, most women in their early forties think the opposite, that they are having signs of menopause when they are really experiencing PMS. When a woman in her forties has gained weight, has lived through a stressful period, or has undergone tubal sterilization, she is a more likely candidate for PMS than for menopause.

## RECOGNIZING THE SYMPTOMS OF PMS

Both women and their doctors have in the past regarded premenstrual syndrome as an inconvenience and "part of being a woman." Rarely did doctors ask women what their symptoms might be. Conversely, women did not think they had a right to complain if their symptoms were mild, and, if symptoms were severe, they were fearful that they might have psychiatric disorders and that their doctors would say, "Sorry, this is not my field, you need a psychiatrist." Inhibition prevailed. There was embarrassment attached to admitting that you felt crazed or clumsy or were wild with food cravings. Women did not want to be ridiculed by their doctors.

Often, the only time a doctor became aware that a patient was really suffering was if she had a dramatic emotional outburst in his office. Then he might begin to pay attention to her symptoms. It has taken a long time for women and doctors to realize that premenstrual syndrome is real. And even today, a woman and her doctor must work as a team to try to diagnose the scope of her condition. Remember, it is estimated that 40 percent of all women between fourteen and fifty years of age experience PMS and that perhaps 10 percent of these women suffer symptoms severe enough to disrupt their daily routines.

The condition is hard to define because symptoms are wide-ranging and women themselves have not known what ailments could be attributed to it. PMS is a medical problem that doctors encourage women to pin down as much as they can before they appear for an office visit. I have always advised women to listen to their bodies, be alert to their symptoms, and to question their doctors about the details of their health problems. With premenstrual syndrome, "listen to your body" is becoming the standard approach. But following an awareness of her body, a woman must find a sensitive physician she can trust, or a reputable health care facility with a staff of medical professionals who compassionately care for patients with premenstrual syndrome.

The best way for a doctor or a clinic to diagnose and treat PMS is through collaboration with the woman who is a patient. Premenstrual syndrome can be divided into different categories, as described in the "Adopting the New Approach" section of Chapter 2, and it is important that a woman and her doctor know which type of PMS she has. To determine all aspects of her condition, a woman must form a partnership between herself and her doctor or counselor. A give-and-take relationship must exist to provide a situation in which a woman can freely discuss her symptoms, ask questions, and be questioned in return. When her symptoms become disturbing, a woman should do two things: organize a menstrual calendar, and write down as much of her menstrual history as she can remember.

By organizing as complete a packet of information as possible, a woman will be joining health care experts in a shared effort to diagnose and treat her condition. Clarifying symptoms is an important step in the process of identifying PMS, but the health partnership between a woman and her doctor becomes even more obvious and necessary in the case of PMS than it does in many other health care problems. A partnership, with concern on both sides, must be established before symptoms can be openly and easily evaluated.

An all-inclusive list of PMS symptoms is difficult to present because every time a "complete" list is compiled, an unexpected symptom appears on a patient's chart. Regardless, an attempt must be made, and what follows is a gathering of the most frequently described, as well as the occasionally appearing, symptoms of premenstrual syndrome. A woman who suspects that she is a sufferer might study this list as she begins to observe her own symptoms:

## THE WIDE-RANGING SYMPTOMS OF PREMENSTRUAL
## SYNDROME

| *Organs or Systems Affected* | *Symptoms* |
| --- | --- |
| Neurological: | Headache |
| | Motor coordination |
| | Migraines |
| | Epilepsy |
| | Vertigo (dizziness) |
| | Fainting spells |
| Psychological: | Irritability |
| | Mood swings |
| | Weeping |
| | Tension |
| | Frustration |
| | Panic |
| | Exhaustion |
| | Aggression |
| | Anger |
| | Lethargy |
| | Depression |
| | Attempted suicide |
| | Assault/Child abuse |
| | Self-inflicted injury |
| | Alcoholic bouts |
| | Drug abuse |
| Respiratory: | Rhinitis (sniffles and runny nose) |
| | Bronchitis |
| | Asthma |
| | Upper respiratory infections |
| Dermatological: | Uticaria (skin rash) |
| | Acne |
| | Boils |
| | Hives |
| | Herpes attacks |

## SYMPTOMS OF PREMENSTRUAL SYNDROME (Cont'd.)

| Organs or Systems Affected | Symptoms |
| --- | --- |
| Orthopedic: | Backache<br>Joint pains<br>Stiffness |
| Muscular: | Muscle tension<br>Edema (water retention)<br>Abdominal pain<br>Muscle cramps (leg cramps, "charley horse") |
| Ophthalmological:<br>(Eye Symptoms) | Conjunctivitis (pink eye)<br>Runny eyes<br>Blackness around eyes<br>Blurred vision |
| Otolaryngorhinological:<br>(Ear, Nose, and Throat Symptoms) | Hoarseness<br>Sore throat<br>Tonsillitis |
| Urological: | Urethritis<br>Cystitis<br>Frequent urination<br>Edema (water retention)<br>Bloatedness |
| Gastrointestinal: | Food cravings<br>Hunger pangs<br>Abdominal swelling |
| Breasts: | Breast tenderness<br>Breast engorgement<br>Fibrocystic breast disease |

The degree to which a woman who is suffering from premenstrual syndrome is sensitive to symptoms may change from month to month and from woman to woman. A woman should only use this list as a basic guide from which she can chart her symptoms on a menstrual calendar. However, she should keep in mind that she may exhibit other forms of PMS than are specified above. For example, some women report that they become accident prone just before their periods. "I get dropsy," one woman told me. "I drop everything I pick up." Other women say they feel extremely sexy when they're premenstrual.

## PMS AND SEX

Dr. Dagmar O'Connor, director of the sex therapy program at St. Luke's/Roosevelt Hospital Medical Center in New York, definitely sees the premenstruum as a positive time for sex. Women often come to her as patients because they are either not interested in sex or they are sexually dysfunctional. "The only time they feel sexual is right before their periods," says Dr. O'Connor. "As they're trying to gain awareness of their bodies and achieve orgasms, they become very clear that this is a time when they're feeling more sexual and they want to take advantage of it." Many of these women achieve their first orgasms during their premenstrual days.

The aggressiveness that is sometimes generated by PMS may cause a woman to initiate sex. "But," as Dr. O'Connor points out, "there may also be a tremendous fight. Then making up may mean making love. For some women, during premenstrual days, there's a release of emotion that's fantastic." These women often say that they do not want to cure their PMS because they like the sexual drive it gives them. This is their choice, of course.

A woman who wants to overcome premenstrual syndrome must be aware of her symptoms and she must chart them on a menstrual calendar to verify the existence of the condition. It has been said that in Europe female opera singers were permitted to wear a red rose on the days that they had their periods and were performing. The rose was a sign to the audience that they were menstruating and that their voices were not in top form. It was believed that hormonal changes caused tonal qualities to change. If each PMS sufferer can define her condition and the appropriate treatment can be gauged, perhaps the idea that the menstrual cycle brings negative side effects can be eradicated.

## THE MENSTRUAL CALENDAR

A doctor who is attempting to diagnose premenstrual syndrome will ask a woman to keep a menstrual calendar for two or three months, so a woman can choose to speed the process by charting her symptoms beforehand. She will be aiding the doctor, but at the same time she will also be giving herself an insight into the intensity of her condition.

A woman may mark her symptoms on a regular engagement calendar, on the calendars provided in the back of this book, or she can use lined paper

# PMS patient

## MENSTRUAL CALENDAR  Month JANUARY 1983

| WK | SUNDAY | MONDAY | TUESDAY | WEDNESDAY | THURSDAY | FRIDAY | SATURDAY |
|---|---|---|---|---|---|---|---|
| **1** | | | | | | | 1 |
| **2** | 2 | 3 | 4 | 5 | 6 | 7 | 8 |
| **3** | 9 | 10 | 11 | 12 Restless Irritable | 13 Insomnia Restless | 14 Insomnia Restless | 15 Depressed Irritable Insomnia |
| **4** | 16 Depressed Irritable | 17 Depressed Irritable | 18 Irritable Depressed | 19 ↑ Hunger Irritable Depressed | 20 Bloated ↑ Hunger migraine Headache | 21 Bloated ↑ Hunger Headache Depressed | 22 Bloated Irritable ↑ Restless Headache |
| **5** | 23 ↓ Dep. ↓ Irrit. | 24 Relief! M | 25 Great M | 26 Great M | 27 Feel Good M | 28 Good | 29 Good |
| **6** | 30 Energetic | 31 Good | | | | | |

The Menstrual Calendar of a PMS Patient: This calendar shows characteristic symptoms of a PMS patient. Note how PMS-related symptoms worsen during the last few days before menstruation, and disappear at the onset of menstruation (marked with an "M" on this calendar). Menstruation for this woman is January 24.

# Not PMS

| WK | SUNDAY | MONDAY | TUESDAY | WEDNESDAY | THURSDAY | FRIDAY | SATURDAY |
|---|---|---|---|---|---|---|---|
| **MENSTRUAL CALENDAR** | | | | | Month **JANUARY 1983** | | |
| **1** | | | | | | | 1 *Binge* |
| **2** | 2 | 3 | 4 | 5 *Depressed* | 6 *Depressed* | 7 *Depressed* | 8 *Dep.* |
| **3** | 9 | 10 | 11 *Binge* | 12 *Binge* | 13 | 14 *Binge* | 15 |
| **4** | 16 | 17 | 18 *Angry* | 19 *Depressed* | 20 | 21 *Headache* | 22 *Headache* |
| **5** | 23 *Backache* | 24 *M* | 25 *M* | 26 *Depressed* *M Binge* | 27 *M* | 28 *M* | 29 *cried a lot* *M* |
| **6** | 30 | 31 *Depressed* *Binge* | | | | | |

*The Menstrual Calendar of a Patient Who Does Not Have PMS:* This calendar shows symptoms that could mistakenly be interpreted as PMS but are not PMS because they do not appear in a cyclic fashion. Also, symptoms show no sign of intensifying before the onset of menstruation, and disappearing as the menstrual flow begins.

and list the days of the month, one line for each day, and rule off three vertical columns for three months. The first marking is made on day one of her menstrual cycle. She writes an "M" on the date that she begins to flow. From that day on she continues to log every physical and psychological feeling that she thinks may be related to premenstrual syndrome. She may note symptoms in longhand or in her own personal shorthand, or she can use the first initial of a symptom, for example, "D" for depression, "W" for weight gain, "T" for tired, to remind her of what she experienced. (See pages 94 and 95.) Basically, the menstrual calendar is a diagnostic tool for remembering what happened during the month, and for calculating whether symptoms intensify before a woman's period and disappear after her menstrual flow ends. Women have found that it helps to use a capital letter when a symptom is severe and a small letter when it is mildly felt.

Symptoms may appear anywhere from two to fourteen days before the onset of menstruation, but sometimes they start a week after menstruation, or exactly on the day of ovulation. A calendar will help a woman assess her pattern.

To be a PMS sufferer, every month a woman must see an unmistakable sympton-free interval of one to two weeks on her calendar. Usually, she will feel well for at least a week after menstraution. This period of good health proves that she has a cyclic problem rather than an ongoing, chronic disorder. Also, as she keeps her calendar and evaluates her symptoms, a woman may notice that her ailments vary in intensity from month to month.

Since a woman ovulates from alternating ovaries, she is subject to different hormonal levels in her body, depending upon which ovary is at work. During a month that the right ovary is responsible for ovulation, a woman may experience a different hormonal balance than she does in a month when the left ovary is in charge. She may have a month when her symptoms are hardly noticeable and then a month of despair. In addition, symptoms, which react to stress, heighten when a woman's personal environment becomes stressful. So symptom fluctuation may be due to alternating ovaries, or stress, or both.

Dr. Katharina Dalton has reported that the psychological symptoms of depression, irritability, and lethargy are present no matter what physical symptoms may arise. Women who have been in extremely depressive, PMS-connected moods have felt so helpless and hopeless during those times that they have attempted suicide. A women should be aware of the depth of her psychological symptoms. Irritability, irrationality, and uncontrollable aggression have been known to manifest themselves to such degrees that women have threatened and abused loved ones, husbands, or children.

Just before and during menstruation, women also have less resistance to infection and they may succumb to respiratory diseases and viruses more than at other times. Women have been admitted to hospitals with meningitis and pneumonia more often during their premenstrual days than at other times. Tolerance for pain is also low during the premenstruum, which is one reason why backaches and joint pains surface. A woman should also realize that when she experiences PMS, her keenness of judgment may not meet her usual standards, her tolerance for alcohol may diminish, and she may be involved in sudden mishaps.

In the past, women who approached doctors with complaints that added up to PMS were handed prescriptions for tranquilizers, medications that never treated the cause of their problems. The goal of this book is to give women who feel that they may have premenstrual syndrome an understanding of the condition and of the techniques to obtain relief. A women can then take her calendar and a record of her menstrual history, as described below, on a visit to a PMS clinic, a women's health center that recognizes PMS, or a progressive doctor and ask to have her condition verified. If she is a sufferer, curing her case of PMS might be a simple matter of vitamin therapy, improved nutrition, and exercise.

### YOUR MENSTRUAL HISTORY

Premenstrual syndrome, as explained in Chapter 3, is influenced by a woman's personal environment, her biological makeup, and her medical history. A woman who is trying to determine whether she is afflicted with PMS can gain a perspective on the scope of her suffering by recording the history of her menstrual cycle. By answering specific questions and describing her menstrual past on paper, she will see, just as her doctor will, whether she is a likely candidate for the condition. In effect, a woman becomes her own doctor when she keeps a menstrual calendar and compiles her menstrual history. With these aids she may even be able to diagnose her premenstrual syndrome herself, before she sees a physician.

A woman should reflect back on the years that she has been menstruating as she sits down to write her menstrual history. If she cannot remember the answers to the questions that follow, she should consult a close family member, her mother or a sister, for other recollections of the status of her health. These questions are meant to serve as springboards to detailed explanations and thoughts. As a woman creates her menstrual history by recalling events and complications associated with her reproductive system, these queries might help to bring forgotten facts to mind:

1. When was your first menstrual period?
2. What is the length of your cycle?

3. Has the heaviness of your period changed over the years?
4. Has the length or regularity of your periods ever changed?
5. Did you ever experience menstrual cramps?
6. Have you ever had an abortion?
7. If you have tried to conceive, have you had fertility problems?
8. Have you ever had anorexia nervosa?
9. Have you ever gained or lost a great deal of weight?
10. Have your menstrual cycles ever become synchronized with those of women with whom you live or work?
11. Have you ever been on birth control pills?
12. If you have ever been pregnant, did you feel great during pregnancy?
13. Have you had complicated pregnancies?
14. Did you ever experience postpartum depression?
15. Have you had gynecological surgery?
16. Have you had a hysterectomy? Were the ovaries removed?
17. Did you have tubal sterilization (were your tubes tied)?
18. Have you ever had an ectopic pregnancy?
19. Did you ever have an ovarian cyst removed?
20. Do you have Stein-Leventhal syndrome or polycystic ovarian disease?
21. Do you have endometriosis?
22. Have you ever had a tubal infection or pelvic inflammatory disease (PID)?
23. Did you experience early menopause?

Of course, every woman's menstrual and reproductive history is her own health experience put into words. When she completes her history, a woman should be able to assess her answers and gain insights into whether she appears to have a hormonal imbalance. If she has suffered many menstrual problems her hormonal secretions may not be exactly correlated, and a lack of hormonal synchronization might lead to hormonal imbalance and cause PMS.

In addition to signaling hormonal imbalance, a woman's menstrual history will also provide a doctor with indications of what might be influencing her PMS. As described in Chapter 3, there are many situations and conditions that affect the severity of premenstrual syndrome. By reviewing Chapter 3, a woman might even be able to detect her particular influences. Anything a woman can do to define her condition will bring her closer to appropriate treatment. In fact, charting her basal body temperature (BBT), as described below, might also benefit her diagnosis.

## HOW THE BASAL BODY TEMPERATURE (BBT) MAY SIGNAL PMS

The level of a woman's basal body temperature after ovulation may help to indicate the presence of premenstrual syndrome. A woman may record her temperature on her menstrual calendar, or she may ask her doctor for the graphlike BBT chart on which she may plot her daily temperature readings.

The time to start recording the basal body temperature is on the first day of the menstrual cycle, which is the first day a woman begins to bleed. When she wakes up in the morning—and every morning without fail—before she has any activity, eats, drinks, or smokes, a woman should take her temperature. An oral reading is fine.

Usually, a woman's morning temperature is 97.5 before ovulation. At ovulation, her temperature either drops slightly or remains the same. A day or two after ovulation, the reading jumps one degree to 98.5, where it remains until immediately prior to menstruation, when it drops. In fact, the first sign of pregnancy is that a woman's temperature stays at the higher level and does not fall.

The BBT is routinely used to evaluate the course of a woman's cycle and her fertility. Progesterone, which appears in the second half, the luteal phase, of the menstrual cycle, is responsible for a woman's elevated temperature. A woman should have two distinct temperature states. During the first half of her cycle, the follicular phase, her temperature should be lower, but in the second half, the luteal phase, she should have a steady, elevated temperature. If a woman does not have two different temperature stages, as shown on page 100, if her temperature after ovulation fluctuates instead of remaining high and even, she may have insufficient progesterone. Progesterone makes a woman's temperature higher, so if the temperature drops after ovulation a hormonal imbalance is clearly indicated. (See page 100.) A low progesterone level is a sign of premenstrual syndrome, and a woman may have found the cause of her symptoms.

To verify her BBT readings, a woman should ask her doctor to conduct blood tests designed to measure hormonal levels. The results of her blood tests will identify as specifically as possible the cause of her premenstrual syndrome.

The medical tests that a doctor can call upon to help him diagnose premenstrual syndrome are described later on in this chapter, but they are really only adjuncts to the home tests and observations that a woman can carry out herself. In the end, a woman's *own diagnostic groundwork* may prove to be just as valuable, or even more important, than the tests that science provides.

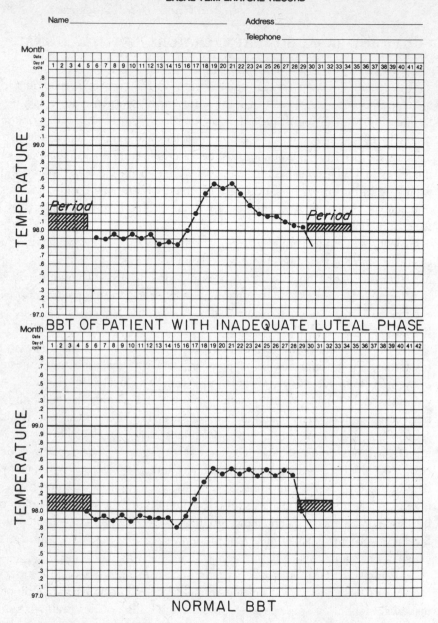

**BASAL TEMPERATURE RECORD**

Name _____    Address _____

Telephone _____

**BBT OF PATIENT WITH INADEQUATE LUTEAL PHASE**

**NORMAL BBT**

*Basal Body Temperature Records:* These figures illustrate basal body temperatures from two different patients. The upper chart illustrates the BBT from a patient with an inadequate luteal phase in which the temperature during the last two weeks of her cycle fluctuates rather than remaining steady and high. This pattern can be seen in women with PMS and in women with infertility problems. The patient might be in need of progesterone treatment. The lower chart illustrates the normal BBT. Note the rise in temperature on day 15 immediately after ovulation, and the persistent high temperature during the luteal phase.

**100**

## HOW TO MAKE AN ACCURATE SELF-DIAGNOSIS

As the stories of Nancy and Pamela at the opening of this chapter show, often it is the loved ones of a woman who is suffering from premenstrual syndrome who are the first to notice that she has symptoms that come and go regularly. However, as more women become aware of PMS, they are personally realizing that their physical and psychological problems are cyclic.

A woman must become sensitive to her bodily functions. If she notices that she experiences recurring monthly symptoms and suspects that she might have PMS, she should carry out the three at-home procedures outlined in this chapter: the menstrual calendar, the menstrual history, and the basal body temperature readings.

By keeping a menstrual calendar for three months, compiling her menstrual history, and charting her basal body temperature, a woman will be gathering evidence that will support or negate her suspicion. She must be careful and disciplined about organizing her menstrual records because they are the foundation for her self-diagnosis.

After reviewing her calendar, history, and BBT readings, as explained in the preceding sections, a woman will have a clear picture of her monthly menstrual patterns. Her records will not be difficult to interpret, and she must trust what she sees. A woman who looks at the facts and concludes that she has PMS may be able to treat herself as competently as she has diagnosed herself. (Methods of self-treatment are discussed in Chapter 5.) However, a woman might want medical verification of her conclusion, or she may have such a severe case of PMS that she feels she needs medical advice on her treatment.

After she has completed two or three months of diagnostic groundwork, she of course would want someone who respects her judgment to take her case. Before methods of self-diagnosis were made known, as they are in this book, women were dismissed by their doctors or referred to psychiatrists. Many PMS patients in my care have told me that in their efforts to find out what was wrong with them they consulted numerous physicians, who never thought to connect their problems with PMS and, in fact, never believed that they had meaningful symptoms.

One woman, the daughter-in-law of a doctor, was ignored by her husband's family for years. They accused her of "having the vapors" and "playing Camille" when what she had was a bad case of PMS. Her marriage was about to disintegrate due to the emotional strain not only of the syndrome but of the put-downs by the people around her. She was on high doses of Valium to control her anxiety. She thought she was crazy and was about to give up the fight to be taken seriously when she heard about PMS.

This woman went to a newly established PMS clinic where she was counseled and taught the self-diagnostic techniques. After returning to the clinic with her completed menstrual calendar, menstrual history, and BBT readings, she underwent blood tests, and her premenstrual syndrome was confirmed. She found relief through the natural treatment method, which is described in Chapter 5, and her attitude about life changed. Even her father-in-law had to admit that "perhaps there was something to this thing called premenstrual syndrome," and that maybe he should have been more tolerant.

If a woman consults a doctor who reveals himself to be unsympathetic, she should immediately seek out a different physician. Health care organizations and clinics listed in Chapter 6 might be able to refer a woman to a physician who recognizes and treats PMS, and some of the clinics are even specifically aimed at caring for PMS patients on the premises. A woman who devotes time, energy, and emotion to working on a self-diagnosis owes it to herself to form a health partnership with a doctor or a counselor who understands the anxiety she has suffered and the courage it took for her to collect her records and ask for help.

## WHAT TO EXPECT FROM A DOCTOR DURING A MEDICAL DIAGNOSIS OF PMS

On the day that a woman consults with a doctor or a counselor about the possibility that she might have premenstrual syndrome, she should remember to bring her menstrual records with her. (In the initial PMS visit, a counselor or a doctor may confer with a woman about her symptoms and health background, but here, for the sake of simplicity, reference is made only to a "doctor.") PMS is probably the only condition for which diagnosis depends more on the timing of symptoms than the symptoms themselves.

With a woman's menstrual calendar, menstrual history, and BBT readings before him, a physician will easily see the pattern of a woman's menstrual cycle, and the fluctuation of her symptoms. A woman might think that if she does not have an exact twenty-eight-day menstrual cycle, she has severe problems. As shown on page 50, the time span of cycles for any given group of women can realistically be plotted on a Bell curve. Twenty-eight days is only the average length of a menstrual cycle. Some women may have their periods every twenty-one days, while others may find that thirty or more days elapse between menstruations. However, women who are on oral contraceptives will have cycles regulated by the pill.

During a consultation in his office, a doctor will interpret a woman's menstrual records and discuss them with her before he begins his internal examination. If a woman seeks a doctor's opinion before she has kept a menstrual calendar or written her menstrual history, he may tell her that he cannot make a proper diagnosis until she has noted her symptoms for two or three months. However, the doctor might elicit a woman's menstrual history during this first visit.

If a menstrual history is being taken by a doctor, a women might look over the twenty-three "menstrual history" questions provided on pages 97 and 98 of this chapter. A doctor should ask the same questions; in fact, it might be helpful if a woman keeps this book open to the questions while she is conversing with her doctor. If she notices that he does not cover all the points listed, she may be able to use the questions as an aid to help her spontaneously contribute to her menstrual history.

Whether or not she arrives with her records, a woman should expect a doctor to talk to her about her symptoms. If he is a concerned physician, he will ask her very personal questions. He may start by inquiring whether anyone in her family has ever experienced PMS, and then he may delve into her private experiences. He may want to know if she has ever attempted suicide, or become physically violent with her husband or children. She may never have told anyone about behavior patterns that she feels are socially unacceptable and she may be embarrassed to reveal herself, but honesty is especially important here.

Premenstrual syndrome can only be correctly diagnosed and treated when all the clinical facts are as precise as possible. A woman must feel that she has a good rapport with her doctor, since she will be asked to express what she may consider to be her hidden secrets, her deepest emotions. If she becomes uptight in any way with the doctor, if she thinks that her openness is thwarted, she should approach a different physician. Since a health partnership is necessary to the diagnosis and treatment of premenstrual syndrome, a woman must sense that she and her physician can have an easy exchange, a free communication.

After your consultation, a doctor will have a good idea about what tests he might want to order for you. However, first he will perform a thorough physical examination.

## THE PHYSICAL EXAMINATION
## FOR MEDICAL DIAGNOSIS OF PMS

At the end of your conversation with the doctor, he will perform a complete physical examination. You'll be asked to urinate so that your bladder is empty and the doctor can have a better chance to examine your organs. Also, you're providing urine to be tested for sugar and protein content, which might indicate upcoming diabetes and kidney problems. You'll change into a gown and wait in an examining room where a nurse will probably weigh you and take your blood pressure before the doctor enters.

The first thing the doctor will do is to feel your neck to be sure that there are no abnormal lymph nodes and that the thyroid gland is not enlarged. An enlargement might indicate a malfunctioning thyroid, and since the thyroid influences the fluctuation of the brain hormones, and the brain hormones affect ovulation and the release of the female hormones, the thyroid must not be overlooked.

Next, a doctor will check your breasts one at a time for lumps. The breast contains several clusters of between ten to one hundred *acini,* glandular sacs grouped around the ducts. These saclike acini are the basic structural unit of the mammary glands. A hormonal imbalance, disturbance in the estrogen/progesterone ratio, may cause the acini and the milk ducts in the breast to expand and form cysts (fluid-filled sacs), which signal fibrocystic breast disease (FBD). Cysts are malleable lumps, always tender to the touch, quite unlike the hard, painless lumps of breast cancer.

If a physician detects any breast abnormalities, he will advise a woman accordingly. If he suspects fibrocystic breast disease, he will ask a woman to monitor her condition through breast self-examination during the course of her next menstrual cycle. For most women, the latter part of the menstrual cycle brings swelling and tenderness of the breast, starting at the time of ovulation and becoming more severe as menstruation approaches. At the onset of the menstrual flow, the normal breast usually returns to its relaxed, less sensitive state. If a breast continues to feel sore and tender after menstruation, a woman may have fibrocystic breast disease.

FBD would indicate a hormonal imbalance, which might be yet another sign that a woman is a candidate for PMS. The doctor should request that you come back at the end of your next menstruation, when your female hormones are at their lowest levels and cystic masses should be diminished. He will then make a more definite evaluation of your condition.

After a doctor finishes examining a woman's breasts, he turns his attention to her abdomen. If he notices any excessive hair growth, he should explain to a woman that she might have an excessive testosterone (male hormone) level. This hormonal imbalance may mean that she has Stein-Leventhal syndrome, with slightly enlarged ovaries, and polycystic ovarian disease, conditions described in Chapter 3. If a woman suffers from Stein-Leventhal syndrome, she may have a hormonal imbalance, which might increase the possibility of premenstrual syndrome.

Upon concluding his external observations, a doctor begins the internal examination. A woman is lying on her back on the examining table with her

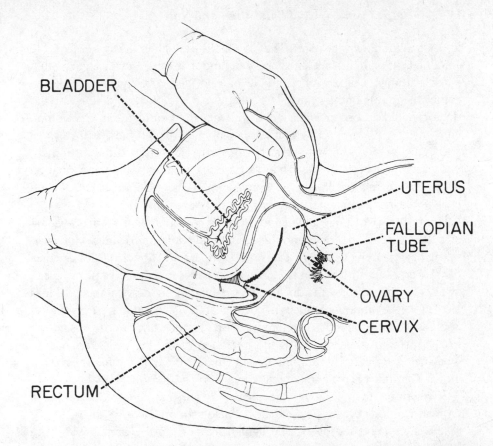

BLADDER

UTERUS

FALLOPIAN
TUBE

OVARY

CERVIX

RECTUM

*The Internal Examination for Medical Diagnosis of PMS:* A doctor examines a woman's internal organs through a bimanual examination while the woman is lying on her back on the examining table with her legs in the stirrups. As pictured, during this examination the doctor inserts the index and middle fingers of one hand into the vagina until he reaches the posterior fornix (the space behind the cervix). His thumb remains on the outside of the vulva, but he should carefully avoid touching the clitoral area. The other hand is resting on the woman's abdomen, and, if she relaxes her abdominal muscles, the doctor shoud be able to palpate the uterus to define its shape and size. He can also determine if the uterus is anteverted, located in the front next to the bladder, as shown in the illustration. If the uterus is retroverted (tilted), it will be pointed downward toward the rectum, which, in the illustration, is located beneath the doctor's internally positioned fingers. The doctor can also palpate the ovaries and tubes (the organs to the right of the uterus) by moving his hands to the side of the uterus. (Reproduced from *Listen to Your Body,* Fireside/Simon & Schuster, Inc., 1982.)

knees bent and her legs apart. The doctor sits on a chair facing her legs. He shines a light on her genital area and examines her outer vulva. Then, with a small instrument called a speculum, he looks inside the vagina and checks the cervix, the mouth of the womb. The speculum comes in various sizes and the doctor should choose the version that's exactly right for his patient. A woman who knows she has a narrow vaginal opening may suggest that he use a small speculum. If a woman is a virgin, he may entirely disregard the instrument and examine her with a swab. If a doctor does use a speculum, it should be warm, and there's nothing wrong with a woman asking her doctor to take the chill off the instrument with a heating pad or hot water.

During the speculum examination, a doctor can only see a woman's vagina and cervix, he cannot peer into the uterus and study her ovaries. However, upon inspecting the cervix, he can see if there are any abnormalities, such as cervical erosions, and he can also tell if a woman is in the middle of her cycle, at or near ovulation, by the quality and quantity of her cervical mucus. He is also aware that abundant mucus might indicate that a woman's estrogen level is excessive and she may therefore have an estrogen imbalance causing her PMS. The Pap smear, which is the next step of the internal examination, while being evaluated for abnormal cells, can also be analyzed for its estrogen index. This index is yet another way of verifying a hormonal imbalance.

A physician then removes the speculum and continues to examine a woman's internal organs bimanually. A doctor can outline the size and shape of the uterus and the ovaries by gently pressing on the organs with both hands. The finger of one hand is placed inside the vagina to steady the organs. The other hand is rested outside the abdomen, and by moving the hand in a circular motion, the doctor can tell if there are any abnormalities such as a retroverted (tilted) uterus, fibroid tumors, or endometriosis.

The entire internal examination should be done slowly and gently, without embarrassment to the doctor or to the woman. A woman should feel free to ask her doctor to explain what he is doing as he is doing it.

• *Deciding to Test Further.* After having taken a medial history and completed a physical examination, a doctor should suggest that a woman keep her menstrual calendar for two or three months, and record her BBT readings, if she has not done so already. If the doctor has not discovered any abnormalities that need special attention, such as fibroid tumors, endometriosis, or ovarian cysts, and a woman's organs are normal, he should make a judgment about further testing.

If he suspects PMS, a doctor should arrange for a woman to have her blood tested when her PMS symptoms are most severe. A woman should be attuned to her menstrual cycle and be able to estimate which of her premenstrual days bring on noticeable suffering. If a woman happens to be in consultation with her doctor during the time that her symptoms are intense, then he should take her blood samples immediately and send them to a laboratory for evaluation. However, if a woman's worst PMS days are in the future, she can make an appointment to return to the doctor's office, or her physician can write down the tests he requires and she can go to a local lab and request the tests herself. If a woman must travel a long distance to her doctor's office, it might be to her convenience to visit a laboratory in her area.

## BLOOD TESTS FOR ANALYSIS OF PMS

People who have been reluctant to believe that PMS is real have been cited in media reports as saying that premenstrual syndrome cannot be specifically diagnosed because blood tests are inconclusive. While it is true that the best way to diagnose PMS is probably through scrutiny of a woman's menstrual calendar and her menstrual history, blood tests can provide a doctor with added information about a woman's hormonal makeup, information that helps create a more accurate diagnosis.

A doctor should order a CBC (a complete blood count), an SMR–12 (an evaluation of a woman's blood chemistry), and hormonal analyses of her blood samples. The selection of a laboratory is very important because one lab may have different test standards than another laboratory, and analyses of data may vary. If blood samples are taken at the right time—when a woman's PMS symptoms are most severe—and her doctor meticulously evaluates the lab reports, blood tests can be a great aid in the diagnosis of premenstrual syndrome.

• *The CBC (Complete Blood Count).* A CBC is an overall evaluation of a woman's white and red blood cells. A doctor should request that any abnormalities in cell counts be reported. If red blood cells are low, for example, a woman may be in a state of hemodilution, which means that she has too much plasma in relation to red blood cells. Hemodilution may be a sign that a woman is suffering from a great deal of water retention. A low blood count may also be a sign of anemia, which may bring on fatigue and depression. An elevated white blood count could indicate an infection somewhere in the body, and might be one reason why a woman does not feel well.

• *The SMR–12 (Evaluation of Blood Chemistry).* Besides indicating whether a woman is suffering any malfunctions in her liver, kidneys, or heart, the SMR–12 will show electrolyte and mineral levels, which may influence the severity of a woman's premenstrual syndrome. The electrolytes, including sodium and potassium, may make a woman's symptoms more pronounced if they are imbalanced, for example, if sodium is high or potassium is low.

The results of the SMR–12 will also be able to tell a doctor whether a woman's calcium level is normal, and what her phosphorous and protein levels are. If blood has been withdrawn while a woman is fasting, the SMR–12 can provide a doctor with his patient's basic glucose level. A low glucose level may mean that a woman is suffering from hypoglycemia, and some patients with hypoglycemia may also be suffering from PMS. A suspicious blood sugar level should be investigated more thoroughly with a glucose tolerance test (GTT), which will determine whether a woman has diabetes or hypoglycemia.

## HORMONAL ANALYSES

Since hormonal imbalance is considered to be the source of premenstrual syndrome, a doctor should request that a woman's blood be analyzed for levels of the following hormones:

• *Prolactin.* Prolactin, one of the hormones released by the pituitary gland, is responsible for the production of breast milk, and it also influences the appearance of breast cysts. Since research has linked prolactin to the presence of premenstrual syndrome, a doctor should study a woman's prolactin level. If prolactin is high, it can be lowered with medication.

• *Thyroid Hormones.* The thyroid gland is involved in stimulating the hypothalamus of the brain, which, in turn, releases the pituitary hormones FSH and LH, which trigger the menstrual cycle. So if a woman's thyroid is underactive, it will not be able to stimulate the brain hormones sufficiently, a proper ovulation will not take place, and an imbalance will occur between estrogen and progesterone. So the hormonal imbalance that could lead to PMS may start with the thyroid.

T3 and T4 tests should be ordered for evaluation of a woman's thyroid function. Even if she only has a slightly low or what is called a "low-normal" thyroid function, it may be enough to diminish her progesterone production to the degree that she has an imbalance of the female hormones. A woman whose tests show low readings may find that she has some relief from her PMS after she takes thyroid medication.

• *FSH (Follicle Stimulating Hormone) and LH (Luteinizing Hormone).* A few days after menstruation has ended, the hypothalamus of the brain sends a hormonal message to the pituitary gland to begin the action of the menstrual cycle. The pituitary gland receives the message and releases the Follicle Stimulating Hormone—FSH—which travels through the blood to the ovaries. FSH triggers estrogen production. Then, about halfway through the cycle, the pituitary reacts to the increased estrogen by sending out the Luteinizing Hormone—LH—which stops the FSH and instigates ovulation. The second half of the menstrual cycle begins and progesterone increases.

FSH, which is arrested by the appearance of LH during the cycle, and LH, which is only high for twenty-four hours at the time of ovulation, should both appear to be at low levels during a woman's premenstruum. FSH and LH are brain hormones related to the production of the female hormones, so if FSH and LH are high during premenstrual days, a doctor should assume that estrogen and progesterone are not in balance. Thus, an analysis of FSH and LH is yet another method of determining whether a PMS-causing hormonal imbalance may exist.

• *Estrogen and Progesterone, the Female Hormones.* Serum progesterone and estradiol (estrogen) levels vary greatly during the menstrual cycle. Readings will often depend upon the phase of the cycle during which the blood tests were taken. In the first half of the menstrual cycle, the follicular phase from menstruation to ovulation, estradiol steadily increases, while progesterone levels remain low. However, in the second half of the menstrual cycle, the luteal phase from ovulation to menstruation, progesterone and estrogen should climb together in a proper balance.

Hormonal levels must be carefully interpreted according to the timing of the blood tests. For instance, the normal value of progesterone during the course of a woman's menstrual cycle may range from .1 to 29 nanograms per milliliter. In the luteal phase, progesterone might be between 5 and 20 nanograms per milliliter. The estradiol level can vary anywhere from 30 to 400 picograms per milliliter during a menstrual cycle, and in the luteal phase might be anywhere from 50 to 150 picograms per milliliter.

A doctor should think more about the ratio of progesterone and estrogen than he does about what might be the "normal" values of these two hormones. In other words, a woman's female hormones should be judged by the way they compare to each other at the moment a blood test was performed, not in how they compare to a laboratory's estimates of normal hormonal levels. If during a specific phase of a woman's cycle her serum progesterone is lower than anticipated in relation to her estrogen, which is higher than expected, then a doctor should consider a possibility of a progesterone/estrogen imbalance. Also, a doctor should take into account that some women have hormonal fluctuations that vary from month to month, depending on which ovary is ovulating. A doctor might choose to perform blood tests a few times during a woman's cycle, and even during different cycles, in order to make comparisons. Some women even have an imbalance of their female hormones that does not clearly show up in the results of their blood tests.

Hormone levels in the bloodstream can be measured, but science has not yet found a way to determine hormonal levels in body tissues, at the level of their hormone receptors. Since estrogen and progesterone receptors exist in tissues, and these receptors affect the body's hormonal content, an incalculable imbalance may be occurring. A physician may decide to treat a woman with hormonal therapy even though he has no exact readings to support his decision. He may feel that her clinical symptoms suggest an imbalance that he is as yet unable to produce on paper.

• *Testosterone, the Male Hormone.* Analysis of the male hormone testosterone does not appear to be important in determining the presence of PMS. However, women who have Stein-Leventhal syndrome, which can be indicated by excessive body hair, might have an elevated male hormone level.

A doctor must be very shrewd in his analysis of hormonal levels. His judgment is extremely important because testing for hormonal levels is not like testing for pregnancy, where there is a definite negative or positive result. The readings of hormonal values, and in fact the results of all blood tests taken for PMS, require careful interpretation. A blood test must be regarded as only one aid that a doctor can call upon to help him confirm a diagnosis of premenstrual syndrome.

## EVERY WOMAN IS DIFFERENT

There is not a defined set of symptoms, appearing on a certain day of the month, that each PMS sufferer shares. Every woman with premenstrual syndrome has her own, personalized PMS profile that becomes apparent after she keeps her menstrual calendar and compiles her menstrual history.

Premenstrual syndrome is an extremely individualized condition. The only experiences common to all sufferers are that the symptoms become more intense during the time between ovulation and menstruation, and that there is a symptom-free interval during each menstrual cycle. A woman with PMS should not expect to find another woman with symptoms quite like hers.

Since the syndrome varies from woman to woman, and even from month to month in the same woman, a PMS sufferer can gain the best understanding of her condition when she forms a health partnership with a doctor or a counselor who cares. A woman's symptoms should be evaluated by the woman herself in collaboration with her doctor. There is always a chance that a physical problem other than premenstrual syndrome may be causing her to feel out of sorts.

If a doctor rules out other health problems and feels that PMS can be diagnosed from the facts that a woman has provided, he may decide against performing blood tests. Blood tests help to determine whether a hormonal imbalance is causing a woman's premenstrual syndrome, and whether hormonal therapy may be appropriate. However, a physician may feel that a woman's clinical symptoms alone provide enough information for him to make a tentative diagnosis and to initiate treatment.

A woman with PMS should always take her personal environment into consideration. Stress, as well as the calming effects of a woman's close relationships, can make a difference in the way she is able to overcome her condition. Relatives and friends must be convinced of the seriousness of the syndrome.

Since many leading physicians now accept PMS as a reality, scientists and doctors are devoting more energy and time to learning how to treat the condition. With knowledge growing every day, there is no need for a woman to believe that there is no cure for this monthly malady. The next chapter will explain how you can begin to conquer PMS right now. You may start undertaking ways to treat your condition by yourself; in fact, self-treatment is sometimes all that is needed. If self-treatment does not seem effective, you can enter into consultation with a physician who can guide you to methods of overcoming the syndrome that has plagued you for so long.

# 5

---

# Modern Treatment of PMS—Next Month Can Be Different

A woman is taking her first step toward overcoming PMS at the moment she realizes she is a sufferer. Awareness leads to proper treatment, but there is a catch. To reach complete relief, a woman must share her awareness with her loved ones.

Everyone in a family is affected when a woman who is someone's wife, mother, daughter, or sister has PMS. Family members, especially young children, react to a woman's premenstrual syndrome, and a woman, in turn, responds to their reactions. While loved ones may be the first to notice a woman's cyclic symptoms, they might still have trouble understanding what she experiences month after month. However, if those close to a sufferer make efforts to grasp the extent of her condition, they will help her treatment immensely.

Following her own awareness of premenstrual syndrome, a woman needs good communication with her family and friends, as well as emotional support from them. A severely afflicted woman and her partner can come closer to comprehending PMS and its effects on their relationship if the two of them seek medical counsel together. By understanding her specific case of PMS, a woman—both by herself and with her mate—will be better able to implement her cure.

Many women can completely eliminate their suffering with communication and support from their loved ones, and modification of nutritional habits and exercise routines. Extreme sufferers might need more involved medical treatment, and it might take months before the appropriate regimen can be found. However, with the information about the complexity and causes of PMS that is now available, almost every woman can be successfully treated and introduced to a life that is free from premenstrual misery.

After diagnosis, as she begins to learn what she can do for herself, and what phases of treatment require medical supervision, a woman must not forget that *communication with her loved ones* is foremost in importance, and essential to her recovery.

## FAMILY COUNSELING

A woman's husband, family, and friends might be more crucial than any medical specialist in helping her to overcome PMS. The people with whom a woman lives and works can provide support and understanding, and reinforce her realization that she is not crazy, that her behavior is the result of a real, hormonally based problem. She should tell her loved ones everything she reads and learns about her condition, and perhaps schedule a special counseling session with her physician or PMS adviser. Modern treatment of PMS emphasizes compassion and rapport between a sufferer and her loved ones, and a physician or counselor should be delighted to answer your questions.

Often families need counseling as much as women themselves. A husband must be able to adjust to his wife's hormonal fluctuations and changing symptoms as she proceeds through the treatment process. He has probably already lived through emotionally chaotic times when he did not know what was happening. Now that he and she both realize that PMS is the problem, he must call upon his patience, sensitivity, and understanding to make the home environment as serene as possible, to reduce the stress and the guilt that can often intensify symptoms.

While a woman is trying to control and cure herself, her man's loyalty and love are extremely important. It may also rest upon the husband/father to help his younger children gain insights into their mother's health crisis and join in mutual supportiveness. Teenage girls should be approached a little differently than the youngsters. These young women might have menstrual cycles timed with their mother's and they might have coinciding, hard-to-manage monthly symptoms, too. During this treatment interval, a mother and her teenage daughter should strive for a loving friendship to enrich their parent/child relationship and to help them conquer what may be a common problem that they share. A teenage boy may not be as attuned to a mother's PMS as his teenage sister is, but he too should be informed and encouraged to show his concern and affection.

Patients often visit my office because a husband, mother, or sister told them about PMS and felt that they might be sufferers. Many women, driven by a fear that they might lose self-restraint and abuse a child or an adult to whom they are close, choose to ask for diagnosis and treatment on their own. Relief comes when women and their loved ones discover that PMS is the reason for a woman's problems and that this condition can be treated.

Once a woman accepts the knowledge of her condition, she must teach her loved ones about PMS through books such as this one, by arranging a private counseling session, or by inviting her family and friends to join her at a PMS support-group meeting, which a number of PMS clinics and women's health organizations sponsor. If a woman's family resists believing that her symptoms are physically based and real, there is no way that she is ever going to improve. Like women who have the postpartum blues, women with premenstrual syndrome need the support, understanding, and encouragement of their loved ones. It is the concern of family and friends that makes treatment effective.

If a woman suspects that her premenstrual syndrome is especially *severe,* she should visit a physician or a PMS adviser at a reputable PMS clinic. On the first appointment, she should bring her husband, or someone close to her, so that he or she will be involved in her discussion with the doctor and hear his evaluation of her condition and his advice about treatment. I always find it a great help for a woman to be supported by an understanding partner. I have witnessed wives and husbands, ready to dissolve their marriages, change their minds after they understand that their problems are rooted in recurring premenstrual syndrome. They are especially inclined to stay together once they hear that the condition can be eliminated through treatment.

During the initial consultation or a special counseling session, a partner, family member, or friend can ask questions that might not occur to you as a patient. For instance, a husband may want to know how your treatment is going to affect your home life, your lovemaking, and other areas of your partnership. A doctor should provide explanations that, while helping to untangle the complexities of this condition, serve as a bridge between two people.

When a woman and her family fully realize that she is suffering from PMS, she must begin to help herself by altering her lifestyle and changing habits and activities that might be heightening her symptoms. With awareness and an understanding of PMS, a woman can take many steps on her own to subdue this syndrome that at times may have seemed to overpower her.

## SUPPORT FROM THE WORKPLACE

If, in addition to support from her family, encouragement in overcoming PMS were provided at the workplace, a woman's determination to conquer the condition would be doubly strengthened. Recognition of PMS is beginning to occur in industry, and the education of employers and employees must be encouraged to continue.

Now that the doctors and nurses who staff the health care facilities at sizable companies are gaining an awareness of PMS, they are starting to notice its effects on women workers. Before PMS was widely accepted as a real condition, a woman who complained of headaches, dizziness, irritability, or general discomfort was usually given medication to ease the pain of menstrual cramps, and she was sent back to work. Today, as one corporate nurse explains, "I'm looking back through my records to see if a woman who comes to me has been in the office with a regular pattern of complaints. Now I'm much more aware of what a woman is talking about, and if she describes the same irritability or depression month after month, I can associate it with PMS. Before, I couldn't have done that. So now, rather than give women something for cramps, I'm trying to advise them about vitamins and exercise."

It is now becoming apparent that the women who have been labeled "trouble" by co-workers or bosses are often PMS sufferers. I regularly hear women who come to me for PMS say that they know they have "bad names" at their offices, because in the past, when they experienced symptoms of PMS, they sometimes lost restraint. They even feel that they have been denied promotions because they have poor reputations. There are other women who have been called "uncooperative" when they really were only suffering from PMS.

By way of comparison, it is interesting to consider how alcoholism has been dealt with in the workplace. When workers are unable to accomplish their jobs because they are alcoholics, they are often excused at first, sometimes others fill in and cover up, but they are not branded. In fact, employers often suggest therapy or treatment programs, AA meetings, and family counseling to problem drinkers. Some businesses may even have work-sponsored treatment programs, and jobs may be guaranteed for *reformed* alcoholics. When male workers are suffering from alcoholism, their male bosses often have compassion. Sometimes men can be easier on men who have problems they understand than they are on women who are suffering in ways that are difficult for them to comprehend. An understanding of PMS must be communicated to the men and women in power so that women who are PMS sufferers can be granted the same nonjudgmental treatment that is offered to workers who are alcoholics.

It is hoped that through women's networks and the distribution of educational material and books employers and employees will become informed about the many facets of PMS. Businesses should be encouraged to provide health information to all supervisors and workers about how PMS may affect women in the workplace. The goal is to create awareness among all people so that no one who is suffering is left untreated. A woman should not be considered a less than ideal worker if she has PMS; instead, she should be commended for recognizing her condition and seeking treatment.

Everyone should aim to eliminate premenstrual syndrome as an issue in the workplace. Women workers might advocate that every woman and man be informed about the symptoms and methods of overcoming the condition. Employers might even conduct educational seminars about PMS and offer referral services through their health care facilities. There is often more understanding given to alcoholics or men who are under pressure or short-tempered on hot summer days than there is offered to women who are enduring PMS, a hormonally based physical condition.

PMS, which can be aggravated by stress, is likely to intensify when women are in highly charged working environments. Women may even quit in frustration and lose jobs that they desperately need. Yet, if a woman received compassionate support from her colleagues in the workplace, she might steadily improve and PMS might become one of those uncontestable issues. Once there were debates about whether women should be allowed to wear pants in the office, but today, what was once controversial is totally accepted. PMS must be accepted, understood, and treated. It is hoped that in the future, women in the workplace will no longer be discriminated against because they have this cyclic, hormonal condition.

## CONQUERING PMS

A woman may be able to manage her PMS by herself, just as she is able to recognize and diagnose the condition. When symptoms are mild, "The Natural Approach to PMS Relief," which comprises a change in a woman's diet, vitamin regimen, and exercise routine, may provide her with an effective way to conquer PMS. In fact, no matter how grave a woman's symptoms are—whether they are hardly noticeable or incapacitating—she should begin her cure with the natural approach, as described later on in this chapter.

A woman who suspects that she has premenstrual syndrome should consult a physician who treats PMS, or a counselor at a reputable PMS clinic. If a woman does not have access to a PMS specialist, she should visit her family doctor or gynecologist. An increasing number of physicians are making sincere efforts to understand the condition and a woman is very likely to find that her own physician can treat her with good judgment.

If she has not already kept a menstrual calendar (see Chapter 4), before her consultation is over, her doctor will ask her to organize a menstrual calendar for two or three months. He will also conduct additional testing. At this time, a doctor should inform a woman about what can be done to reduce her symptoms by the natural approach. If after a couple of menstrual cycles, the natural approach does not alleviate her symptoms and her blood tests indicate a severe hormonal imbalance, medical treatment designed to correct the imbalance should be started. This treatment, described in this book as "The Medical Approach to PMS Relief," should be initiated in combination with the natural regime.

The *medical approach,* which includes hormonal therapy, is suggested for women who find that PMS is affecting the quality of their lives by creating symptoms that harm their personal relationships and prevent them from functioning normally. When the results of a woman's blood tests are evaluated, a doctor might find a hormonal imbalance that may prompt him to advise the medical approach for a woman. There is also the possibility that a woman has begun self-treatment and found no relief. Her case might be so severe and her suffering so terrible that a doctor might start the medical approach even before all the blood tests are completed. Then, when the results of the blood tests are reported, he might modify the treatment accordingly. The decision to proceed with immediate medical treatment is often made when a doctor is faced with a health problem that he thinks might worsen during a wait for test results. For example, when a woman has a bladder infection, a doctor will begin treatment immediately if he judges that it would be detrimental to her health to wait for the urine culture and sensitivity test. When the urine analysis finally is reported, he might change her medication if test results show that she is not receiving the most effective therapy. In relation to PMS, the natural approach should be continued even if the medical treatment is altered. In fact, the natural approach should always be the first method chosen when an attempt to relieve PMS is made.

By looking back to the "Adopting the New Approach" section of Chapter 2, a woman will see that premenstrual syndrome can be divided into four separate categories according to her symptoms. A woman should scrutinize the symptoms on her menstrual calendar and review the four categories—PMT–A (anxiety, irritability, nervous tension), PMT–H (weight gain, abdominal bloating, fluid retention), PMT–C (food cravings, hypoglycemic symptoms), PMT–D (depression, withdrawal, lethargy, confusion, suicidal feelings)—to determine which division best describes her particular group of symptoms.

By understanding her individual syndrome, she will see that in her case certain treatments should be emphasized more than others. For example, if she feels that her problem is PMT–A (anxiety, irritability, nervous tension), methods of stress reduction may have greater priority than the lessening of her salt intake. For a woman with PMT–H (weight gain, abdominal bloating, fluid retention), salt reduction would be especially important. Still, no matter what form of premenstrual syndrome a woman is trying to control, all facets of the natural approach should be included in her treatment program. PMS is a systemic condition that can only be overcome with a mind/body treatment in which the entire woman is considered, not just individual symptoms.

However, it is important that the whole family understand whatever treatment is instituted and that they participate and help her stay on her course of recovery. The support of a woman's loved ones is essential to her triumph over PMS.

## The Natural Approach to PMS Relief

Many women with PMS say that they become obsessed with food cravings during their premenstruum. Women desire salty foods, sugars, or starches; they have one or a combination of cravings. "The Natural Approach to PMS Relief" aims to curb food cravings through nutritional techniques and vitamin and mineral supplementation. Alterations in diet also help to reduce fluid retention and psychological symptoms, since the release of the brain's hormones and neurotransmitters seems to be influenced by vitamin and mineral levels.

Stress also may inhibit or activate hormonal secretions in the brain that in turn may affect hormonal flows in other parts of the body and bring on PMS. So stress reduction through exercise and meditation is another ingredient in the natural approach. Since every woman's body is unique and each case of premenstrual syndrome is singular, a woman, either alone or with her doctor, must evaluate her symptoms and decide which segment of the natural approach is most meaningful to her.

To plan her treatment, a doctor should first take a woman's diet history, or she can organize her diet history herself. It is important that a woman understand what she is doing before she moves on to what must be done. Among the questions a woman should ask herself are:

1. How much do you salt your foods?
2. Do you eat balanced meals at regular intervals or do you starve yourself all day only to eat a large meal at night?

3. How often do you eat sweets? Every day? Several times a month? Hardly ever?
4. Do you eat green vegetables regularly?
5. Are fresh fruits included in your diet?
6. Are you taking vitamin supplementation?
7. Are you overweight or underweight?

A woman should also question her exercise routines and ask herself how often she is physically active. Then, after reviewing her answers, a woman will probably have an idea, even before her doctor tells her, which nutritional and lifestyle habits might be improved. If her PMS symptoms are mild, a woman should begin self-treatment with the natural approach after studying the method as it is described below.

## PLANNING THE NATURAL APPROACH

PMS has been found to disappear when women have made nutritional changes in their diets. However, a woman must remember that different food groups, vitamins, and minerals affect different symptoms. So in order to plan a nutritional program that will eliminate her particular problems, a woman must learn where, in her case, changes would be most effective.

## SALT INTAKE

Salt, or sodium chloride, maintains the fluid level in a woman's body; however, a hormonal imbalance (excessive estrogen or an imbalance in the aldosterone system) may escalate the internal salt content. Then, the excess salt will cause fluid retention, since salt binds water. Body tissues, including the brain membrane, will swell. Eventually, the brain swells and its membrane stretches to the limitations of a woman's skull. The brain would swell more and more if it were not trapped inside the skull, but because it is trapped, its expansion is held back. The water pressure builds inside the head, irritating the brain's nerve endings. As a result, a woman experiences headaches, dizziness, agitation, nervousness, and confusion. In addition, she might have weight gain and bloatedness. Yet all these symptoms might be diminished if the body's salt content were reduced.

If a woman is experiencing the symptoms described above, or she is a PMS sufferer with a noticeable salt craving, she must begin to control her salt intake to prevent fluid retention. Hermien Lee, a registered dietician and nutritionist in private practice in Beverly Hills, has counseled hundreds of women who have wanted to prevent the weight gain and bloatedness they experience during their premenstrual days. Ms. Lee's advice—which is in accordance with what I tell my patients—is to stay away from salty foods such as cured meats, salty snacks, pickles, sauerkraut, and salts with spices, such as garlic salt. If a woman wants to spice her foods, she might use powders and peppers, which only have a minimal amount of salt, or salt substitutes that are currently on the market. The best method, of course, is the no-salt approach, no salt in cooking or at the dinner table.

Sometimes there is hidden salt in the foods a woman eats. There is salt in most carbonated sodas. Unless a woman purchases the new salt-free kind of club soda, she will be getting more salt than she realizes, since ordinary club soda contains 241 milligrams of sodium. Perrier water, which is another sparkling drink, has only 14 milligrams of sodium, and Poland Spring water a mere 4 milligrams. Obviously, it is most beneficial to have Perrier or Poland Spring water, which a woman may drink with a wedge of lemon for flavoring. Tap water may not be a salt-free alternative because in some areas the sodium content in tap water is high.

A woman can also monitor the salt content in packaged foods. Ingredients in frozen and canned foods are listed in order of quantity, with the foods in highest content appearing first. A woman should always check labels for the ingredients of the foods she buys, and she should select foods with no or low salt. In fact, if possible, it is best to buy fresh fruits and vegetables, which a woman herself can prepare salt-free.

The elimination of salt alone has helped many PMS sufferers reduce their bloatedness, premenstrual irritability, and headaches. Thus, it is specifically important that a woman begin a low-or-no-salt diet during the two weeks preceding her period, when PMS symptoms are usually at their worst.

If a woman still is suffering from fluid retention, diuretics might be helpful in eliminating excess fluid, but they never cure PMS symptoms. Diuretics do not rid the body of the intracellular fluid and sodium that bring on certain PMS symptoms.

## CARBOHYDRATES (SUGARS AND STARCHES)

During the last half of the menstrual cycle, either an imbalance in the release of the brain's hormones and neurotransmitters, an imbalance in the female hormones estrogen and progesterone, or a combination of the different hormonal imbalances triggers a carbohydrate craving in the woman who is suffering from premenstrual syndrome. As Dr. Guy E. Abraham (see Chapter 3) has reported, cells bind insulin and create a high insulin level in the body during the last half, the luteal phase, of the menstrual cycle. This higher insulin level might be caused by one or a combination of the hormonal imbalances mentioned above. At any rate, a high insulin level makes the body's blood sugar fall more rapidly. So a woman with premenstrual syndrome who finds herself with a carbohydrate craving is already likely to have a high insulin/low blood sugar ratio, which means that she might go into a hypoglycemiclike tailspin if she tries to quell the craving by eating a concentrated amount of sugar. The sugar will go right into her bloodstream, her already high insulin will soar, and make her already low blood sugar plummet. This hypoglycemic attack, which usually occurs thirty to sixty minutes after a woman eats sugar in high concentration, will result in extreme fatigue. If a woman continues to eat refined sugar, she will continue to have persistent low-blood-sugar attacks, and they will lead to headaches, depression, agitation, and irritability.

As *The New York Times*'s health columnist, Jane Brody, explains in *Jane Brody's Nutrition Book:* "Insulin overshoot, as doctors call the overproduction of insulin in response to a sugar load, happens to some extent to everyone who consumes a concentrated dose of sugar, especially between meals. It's probably an evolutionary hangover from our early days as a species when the only sources of sugar in the human diet were fruits and vegetables, which come into the body diluted by other digestible nutrients plus water and fiber. The body was not designed to handle sugar in concentrated forms, such as in a piece of cake or candy bar."*

Rather than eating foods that contain concentrated amounts of sugar, a woman should turn to natural carbohydrates. *Natural carbohydrates* are found in fresh fruits and vegetables, whole grains, and beans. These foods include sugars, or *simple* carbohydrates, and starches, or *complex* carbohydrates. *Refined carbohydrates* have been processed out of natural foods and added in high concentration in foods that would not normally have them. Refined sugar and refined flour have refined carbohydrates; therefore, foods such as white bread, pies, cakes, candies, and pasta, which are made with refined sugar and flour, are introducing a too-high concentration of carbohydrates—excessive sugar and starch—into the bloodstream. The impact of a concentrated amount of sugar cannot be overemphasized. The skyrocketing insulin and plummeting blood sugar that result can bring on severe PMS symptoms.

During the last half of her menstrual cycle, a woman can prevent carbohydrate cravings by eating small amounts of food at regular intervals, food that will keep her blood sugar level steady. If a woman allows more than three or

*Jane Brody, *Jane Brody's Nutrition Book* (New York: Bantam, 1982), p. 128.

four hours to go by without eating anything, her blood sugar may drop to the point of causing an extreme sugar craving that when satisfied brings on the depression, tenseness, agitation, and headaches she is trying to overcome.

A woman with PMT–C food cravings and hypoglycemic symptoms should be sure to eat at approximately three-hour intervals in order to keep her blood sugar steady. She should avoid foods with refined carbohydrates and eat meals and snacks that include protein and natural carbohydrates. A woman may choose from cheese, yogurt, nuts, sunflower seeds, eggs, her favorite fruits and vegetables, and unrefined whole grain products, which contain more nutrients than sugary sweets. (A twenty-four-hour nutritional program, an example of an ideal eating day during the premenstruum, is presented in "The PMS Diet" in this chapter.)

When it comes to consuming carbohydrates, nutritionist Hermien Lee, who is also the author of *The Spot Reducing Diet: A Beverly Hills Nutritionist Tells You How to Lose It Where You Want To,* * suggests that at least an ounce of protein be eaten with a carbohydrate. "Never a carbohydrate without a protein!" she says, because proteins take longer to enter the bloodstream and convert into glucose. Carbohydrates enter the bloodstream rapidly and create a demand for insulin to be used in glucose conversion. The insulin climb then may cause a drop in blood sugar, which in turn triggers a PMS mood swing. If, for example, an apple or an orange is eaten with a piece of cheese, which is a carbohydrate paired with a protein, the cheese will temper the effect of the fruit, insulin production will be less dramatic, and the blood sugar will not descend to the symptom-causing level.

The carbohydrate/protein combination or protein alone, eaten at regular intervals, is a method of curbing PMS food cravings. However, there may be a time when a PMS sufferer forgets to eat at regular intervals and becomes overwhelmed by a carbohydrate craving. She may also feel a depression coming on. In this instance, consuming a natural carbohydrate without protein may be beneficial. As reported in Chapter 3, MIT researchers have linked the brain chemical serotonin, which is a mood regulator, to carbohydrate cravings. What a woman experiences as a carbohydrate craving may be the brain's way of increasing its supply of serotonin. The amino acid tryptophan is essential to the manufacture of serotonin, and when a woman consumes carbohydrates she is helping tryptophan to reach the brain, where it is needed to produce serotonin.

Dr. Judith J. Wurtman explains in *The Carbohydrate Craver's Diet*† that carbohydrates must be *eaten alone* to calm the craving and start tryptophan

---

* Hermien Lee, *The Spot Reducing Diet* (New York: Coward-McCann, 1983).

† Judith J. Wurtman, *The Carbohydrate Craver's Diet* (Boston: Houghton Mifflin, 1983).

on its journey through the bloodstream to the brain. According to Dr. Wurtman, if a protein is consumed with a carbohydrate, the other amino acids in the protein will become obstacles to the tryptophan and inhibit its passage to the brain.

Once a carbohydrate craving has surfaced, a woman might eat a natural carbohydrate, such as an apple or green beans, to promote tryptophan and serotonin production. When an adequate serotonin level is reached, this neurotransmitter will send out a signal that stops the craving.

However, at the outset, when a woman is working to keep her blood sugar from drastically fluctuating and producing a craving, she should eat the carbohydrate/protein combination, or protein alone, at regular intervals. A woman should choose natural carbohydrates and protein foods such as fish and chicken, which are lower in fat and calories than red and processed meats. A hard-boiled egg is high in protein and contains only seventy-five calories.

Naturally, if a woman has an extreme craving for something sweet, there may be nothing that can satisfy her but a refined-sugar treat. A tiny piece of cake or a few bites of a candy bar will not be detrimental to her health if she eats slowly and does not go beyond this limit. By savoring a small portion of a sweet snack, a woman can calm a craving more efficiently than she could if she ate a whole serving quickly.

## FLUID INTAKE

A woman who experiences edema (swelling due to fluid retention) throughout her body, especially around her joints, limbs, and abdomen, should limit her fluid intake during the seven days that precede her menstrual flow. She should drink no more than four glasses or cups of fluid a day. Her bloatedness is a sign that the salt content in her body has escalated and that the increased salt is binding water. Normally, fluids are excreted through the kidneys, but when a woman is edematous due to PMS, her salt content causes fluid to be absorbed by body tissues before it passes through her system.

It is important to remember that the brain, which is swelling along with other parts of the body, is causing tension, irritability, and headaches to emerge along with the edema. Scientists involved in researching premenstrual syndrome have suggested that women who tend to bloat or gain weight before menstruation should limit their fluid intake, but women without these symptoms should not be concerned about changing their habits.

• **Caffeine.** Coffee, tea, cola, and chocolate drinks all contain caffeine. Caffeine stimulates the brain, which in turn affects the central nervous system, the activity of the heart and circulatory system, and coordination and respiration. By changing a woman's metabolic rate, caffeine also creates an internal situation in which insulin increases, blood sugar drops, and a hypoglycemiclike attack occurs. Whether or not she is a PMS sufferer, a woman who consumes several caffeine-containing beverages a day might develop caffeine-induced food cravings.

A woman whose PMS symptoms include food cravings along with depression, tenseness, agitation, and headaches has a higher-than-average susceptibility to the effects of caffeine, and she should avoid it on heightened PMS days. In fact, many women find that caffeine tends to worsen PMS symptoms in general. No matter what types of premenstrual syndrome a woman has, she would be wise to switch to decaffeinated coffee, caffeine-free teas, and no-caffeine carbonated beverages during her premenstruum. There is only one occasion on which caffeine may be considered beneficial. For the woman whose PMS includes fluid retention, a single cup of light coffee or tea might act as a diuretic and reduce her bloatedness.

• **Alcohol.** Women who have premenstrual syndrome have a decreased alcohol tolerance. Some women have actually discovered that they have PMS when they realized that they used to be able to drink more than one glass of wine with dinner, and suddenly, one glass made them feel slightly intoxicated. A woman who is a PMS sufferer cannot tolerate liquor as well during her premenstruum as she does during other times of the month, particularly if fluid retention is one of her symptoms. In fact, in a 1971 survey that appeared in the *Archives of General Psychiatry,* 67 percent of menstruating female alcoholics linked their drinking patterns to their menstrual cycles. In a startling revelation, 100 percent of the women questioned admitted that their drinking problems had either started or intensified during their premenstrual days.

This sensitivity to alcohol, in combination with other PMS symptoms such as diminished motor coordination and reduced self-control, may lead to accidents. A woman should be alert to her changed capacity for liquor, and she should monitor her social drinking. Only one cocktail or glass of wine may be enough to make her feel the effects of PMS intoxication. It is wise for a woman to cut down on or, better, eliminate alcoholic beverages during the premenstruum. Also, to prevent PMS symptoms from worsening, a woman should avoid mixing drinks or combining hard liquor and wine. Another important rule is: Never drink on an empty stomach. If a woman must drink, she should eat a small protein snack such as nuts or cheese, or canapés made with meat, fish, or poultry, since food tempers the effects of alcohol. Still, the best advice of all is to stop drinking when PMS symptoms are due to appear.

You may be a woman who is extremely susceptible to the influence of alcohol, and there is no reason for you to risk your well-being.

## THE PMS DIET

Using the information in this "Natural Approach to PMS Relief," a woman who analyzes and understands her specific case of premenstrual syndrome should be able to see how nutritional changes may help her overcome her symptoms. Her daily diet during the luteal phase of her menstrual cycle should be designed with the goal of eliminating her PMS symptoms. A nutritional program must be supplemented with daily doses of vitamins and minerals as well as methods of stress reduction, but before examining these other regimens, a woman should contemplate how she might revise her eating habits.

Nutritionist Hermien Lee has provided a sample day of good eating for PMS sufferers. This one-day menu is simply a means of giving a woman an idea of how she may reconstruct her eating patterns. The balanced diet offered in this plan would benefit the health of any woman every day of the month. Ms. Lee emphasizes that the well-balanced diet she has presented is, more than anything else, an example of a good nutritional program. The menu is low-calorie, and if the program is strictly followed, a woman will not gain weight, since she will stay well within 1,500 calories a day. However, Ms. Lee is more concerned that women recognize this diet for its nutritional value than for its specific calorie count. Ms. Lee suggests that all her clients, men and women, PMS sufferers or women who never experienced the syndrome, follow this type of plan for weight control and good health.

The last half of the menstrual cycle is the time when PMS sufferers must be most careful about the kinds and quantities of the foods they eat. All portions should be well-balanced and small. Women would be increasing their ability to overcome their symptoms if they incorporate their PMS diets into their lives. With her particular syndrome in mind, a woman should carefully study Ms. Lee's day of good eating, and using this one-day menu as a basic plan, design a diet to conquer her symptoms. It cannot be overemphasized that the PMS diet that helps a woman find relief from her symptoms in the last half of her menstrual cycle would maintain her health and vitality if she followed it every day of her life.

## PMS RECOVERY PLAN—A DAY OF GOOD EATING

A woman should use this food plan as a guide. Information on beverages appears in the preceding "Fluid Intake" section.

• **Breakfast.** If your body does not need food until later on in the day, you can postpone this early-morning meal; you might want to make breakfast a late-night snack. However, after awakening, it is important that a PMS sufferer not allow too many hours to pass before eating some food, such as a carbohydrate/protein combination, or she may experience a severe drop in her blood sugar level.

For a woman who begins her day with breakfast, Ms. Lee suggests an orange or a grapefruit half. No juice in the morning. One glass of orange juice has the sugar of three oranges. Such a highly concentrated amount of sugar may cause an insulin rush and a drop in blood sugar. Also, since vitamin C is lost when it is exposed to the air, juice rapidly loses its vitamin content.

Since Ms. Lee recommends that a carbohydrate never be eaten without a protein, an orange or grapefruit half should be followed by an egg, or one ounce of partially skimmed milk cheese such as mozzarella cheese, or The Laughing Cow green label cheese. The protein may also be a third of a cup of low-fat cottage cheese, or a third of a cup of low-fat plain yogurt, or a tablespoon of peanut butter (prepared as described in the "Between Meals" section) on a slice of whole-wheat or rye bread. A woman may have two slices of whole-grain bread during the day, either at breakfast or at other times. If she prefers her whole grains in cereal, of the popular brands she may choose a half cup of either Shredded Wheat, Puffed Wheat, Puffed Rice, oatmeal, or Wheatena, each of which has less than 5 percent sugar. She should combine her cereal with a half cup of skim or nonfat milk.

• **Lunch.** A woman who did not have an egg at breakfast may choose to have a two-egg vegetable/cheese omelette. A salad featuring either tuna, chicken, turkey, or cold seafood such as shrimp or crab, with cucumbers, tomatoes, spinach, lettuce, or other vegetables, is also a possibility. An accompanying dressing may be made by mixing to taste: tomato juice, Dijon mustard, lemon juice, and garlic. Also included in the dressing are: two chopped hard-boiled egg whites, capers, onion, and chopped pimento. When in a restaurant, where she has no opportunity to make a dressing, a woman may order French, Russian, or Italian dressing on the side and use what Ms. Lee calls "the fork prong" method. A woman may dip her fork into the dressing and then into the salad, thereby getting flavor without too many of the fattening ingredients. (Note: At some PMS clinics, counselors suggest that women create salad dressings with safflower oil, which contains beneficial linoleic acid, vinegar, and spices. Safflower oil, however, is high in calories and a weight-conscious woman might want to limit her intake to not more than two teaspoons of this oil at a time.)

If a woman did not have bread at breakfast she may like a sandwich with sliced turkey, tomato, lettuce, onion, pickle, and mustard on two pieces of rye bread. It's important to drain the salt from the pickle by soaking it in cold water before including it in the sandwich. There should not be any salt or salted flavorings on the sandwich. In fact, a woman who has PMS fluid retention should beware of salt and choose the no-salt alternative as much as possible. Although the avoidance of salt is not as crucial for women with other symptoms, they still should strive for salt-free diets.

• **Between Meals.** Women with PMS should remember to eat food at three-hour intervals to keep their blood sugar steady. Ms. Lee recommends carbohydrate/protein combinations such as a serving of fruit with a third of a cup of low-fat plain yogurt, or a third of a cup of low-fat cottage cheese, or an ounce of partially skimmed milk cheese. Peanut butter may also be a protein selection. A woman could buy old-fashioned peanut butter and pour off the oil by folding a paper towel into quarters and placing the towel on top of the peanut butter, between the peanut butter and the lid. Screw the lid on the jar with the paper towel inside. Turn the jar upside down to allow the oil to drain onto the towel. Change the towel when it is saturated. The peanut butter is ready to eat when it is dull and hard, which is usually in about twenty-four hours. If the peanut butter is shiny and hard, it can be patted dry with a towel. After twenty-four hours, with the oil drained, the peanut butter will be thick and much lower in calories. A woman can then slice half a banana lengthwise, spread a tablespoon of peanut butter along the sliced side, and rejoin the banana to create a peanut-butter-and-banana sandwich, which she can wrap in aluminum foil and freeze. Between meals, frozen peanut-butter-and-banana is an imaginative carbohydrate/protein snack.

• **Dinner.** A portion of lean meat, fish, or poultry can be served with a small baked potato, or two slices of whole-grain bread (if a woman has not eaten any bread or cereal during the day), a salad or a hot vegetable, and fruit for dessert. Although opinions differ, green leafy vegetables, asparagus, and alfalfa sprouts are generally accepted as natural diuretics. A woman who is suffering from fluid retention might want to select these vegetables to help reduce her symptoms.

Ms. Lee recommends pumpkin pudding as a creative all-purpose food. A half-cup of pumpkin pudding stands as a vegetable, while a whole cup may be considered the fruit dessert. Here's how to make the pumpkin pudding: Beat two egg whites until they're stiff. Add the contents of a large can of pumpkin filling. Mix in the spices listed in the pumpkin pie recipe on the can, but do not add butter or sugar. Remember, only include the spices. Then add the contents of an envelope of Equal, a new sugar substitute, and vanilla. Beat the ingredients until they're smooth, spoon the mixture into a small casserole dish, and bake it in an oven set at 350 degrees. The pudding should bake until the top turns brown, which is usually from 20 to 25 minutes.

"Most hunger is mouth hunger, not stomach hunger," says Hermien Lee. Many women eat to calm an anxiety such as the anxiousness that might arise from PMS. A woman must limit her intake and remember that she only needs *small amounts* of food at regular intervals during her premenstruum. Also, she should combine her nutritional program with the methods of stress reduction that are described in this chapter. Eating should not be used as a stress-reliever or an antidepressant.

## MINERALS AND VITAMINS

The minerals that have been found to minimize the severity of various PMS symptoms are calcium, magnesium, zinc, iron, and the electrolyte potassium. The B vitamins and vitamins D, E, A, and C are also important to the body's internal balance and they, too, can diminish the intensity of PMS.

As part of the natural approach, a woman may take a full course of mineral and vitamin supplementation, or she may choose to add only those minerals and vitamins that apply to the treatment of specific symptoms. The minerals and vitamins should be taken every day, but dosages should be increased, as explained in the individual sections below, during the last half of the menstrual cycle or when PMS symptoms appear.

• **Calcium.** The mineral calcium is naturally present in milk and milk products, sardines, mustard and turnip greens, soybeans, raspberries, and citrus fruits. However, people often do not eat these foods in the quantities necessary to maintain adequate calcium levels in their bodies. In addition, women alone are subject to a PMS calcium problem.

Approximately ten to fourteen days before menstruation, the calcium blood level in PMS sufferers tends to decrease. This drop can bring on a calcium deficiency that results in insomnia, headaches, muscle cramps, nervousness, bloatedness, abdominal/menstrual cramps, and pelvic pain. A woman who is suffering from any of these symptoms, particularly cramps and pelvic pain, should take calcium, but always in combination with magnesium, since the two minerals are bound in the body, and taking calcium alone can bring on a magnesium deficiency. (Also see "Vitamin D" for its relation to calcium.)

Calcium is best taken in the form of calcium gluconate tablets, 500-milligrams each. Magnesium is usually taken in milligram tablets equaling half the dosage of the calcium supplements. A woman should take one calcium gluconate tablet daily, and two tablets during the fourteen days preceding her menstrual flow.

If a woman is suffering from severe uterine cramping during her premenstruum, she might take one 500-milligram calcium gluconate tablet with magnesium every two hours, but she should not consume more than six tablets a day. If one tablet every two hours does not bring relief, then she should take two tablets every two hours, still not exceeding six tablets a day, until her cramps are gone. Recently, a patient of mine who suffered from uterine cramps and waves of pelvic pain that intensified a few days before her period was advised to take calcium gluconate tablets. She took only five tablets with magnesium on the first day of her symptoms, two tablets on the second day, and by the third day her cramps had disappeared without any other treatment.

An oversupply of calcium is usually excreted in urine and stools, so a healthy woman should not worry about taking calcium supplements to alleviate her symptoms. A woman who has kidney stones, or other conditions that require a careful monitoring of her calcium intake, should confer with her doctor before taking this supplementation. A series of blood tests might scientifically verify a woman's deficiency, but if she finds relief with supplementation, she can be sure that a calcium deficiency exists and there is no reason for her to undergo further testing.

• *Magnesium.* Nuts, soybeans, green leafy vegetables such as spinach, chard, kale, and beet tops, seeds, and whole grains are rich in magnesium. The green leafy vegetables provide their supply of magnesium if they are eaten raw or cooked in a small amount of water that is not discarded. Chocolate, too, is magnesium-rich, but chocolate also contains caffeine, which worsens PMS.

Symptoms of a PMS-induced magnesium deficiency are nervousness, insomnia, muscle cramps, abdominal/menstrual cramps, and pelvic pain, essentially the same symptoms as a calcium deficiency. Magnesium and calcium go hand in hand, so even if magnesium is increased, it should remain at half the extra calcium intake. In other words, magnesium is taken at half the dosage of calcium, and if magnesium is increased, calcium should be increased twice as much.

As mentioned before, if a woman has kidney stones or other problems of the excretory system, she should ask her doctor if it is all right for her to supplement her diet with extra calcium and magnesium. Otherwise, in order to curb PMS, a woman should take one 500 milligram tablet of calcium gluconate a day along with about 250 milligrams daily of magnesium, and she should increase her intake to two daily calcium gluconate/magnesium tablets during the last half of her menstrual cycle.

• *Zinc.* Shellfish are dependable sources of zinc. In varying degrees, this mineral is also found in meat, poultry, eggs, milk, and whole grains. Zinc, which is present in all human tissue, is necessary to successful enzyme activity within the body. Zinc is also at the core of our being. Without zinc, RNA and

DNA, components of the nucleus of each body cell, do not develop properly. A zinc deficiency during pregnancy might inhibit proper growth of an unborn's brain.

Also, a zinc deficiency may lower a woman's resistance to infection, contribute to infertility, and impede her body's healing process. During the premenstruum, a zinc deficiency might lead to irritability, depression, and other PMS symptoms such as headaches and nervousness.

To treat her PMS, a woman should take 30 milligrams of zinc each day, and increase her intake to 50 milligrams during her premenstruum. Zinc can be taken along with calcium and magnesium but it should not be taken with iron. When zinc and iron are combined, the two minerals prevent each other's absorption into the bloodstream.

• **Iron.** The best sources of iron are organ meats such as liver and kidney, apricots, and eggs, or, more precisely, egg yolks. Other iron-containing foods are meat, yeast, wheat germ, whole grains, blackstrap molasses, and potatoes. A woman who bleeds heavily during her periods may be a candidate for iron deficiency.

If a woman is iron-deficient she will experience weakness and fatigue due to anemia. Her tiredness can be so overwhelming that she does not even have the strength to exercise and combat her PMS. In fact, the symptoms of premenstrual syndrome may seem to increase in severity because she is unable to fight them. Then depression might ensue.

A woman who recognizes weakness and fatigue, particularly as part of her premenstrual syndrome, should take iron in the form of ferro-sulphate or ferro-gluconate, 300 milligrams three times a day, every day of the month. If a woman prefers, she may take a single long-acting iron capsule each day. Some women have even found that one prenatal vitamin with iron is enough to increase their energy and their blood count.

Iron should be taken in combination with vitamin C, which aids in the body's iron absorption. Thus, the designated iron intake with 1,000 to 1,500 milligrams of vitamin C each day should help to strengthen a woman and diminish the intensity of her symptoms. If iron supplementation seems ineffective against PMS, a woman might have anemia due to the malabsorption of iron or a vitamin $B_{12}$ deficiency. Whatever the reason, if extra iron is not improving her health, a woman should consult her doctor or PMS counselor to confirm her deficiency through blood tests. A severe iron deficiency should be medically treated.

• **Potassium.** If a woman's diet includes bananas, oranges or orange juice, dried fruits, or unsalted nuts she is supplying herself with potassium, a mineral that is considered an *electrolyte*. Since potassium helps to regulate fluid retention, a woman who feels bloated may have too much body fluid due to a potassium deficiency. The deficiency may exist either because a woman is taking diuretics and excreting an excessive amount of this electrolyte, or because she is not eating enough potassium-rich foods.

When potassium is lacking, sodium and fluid are retained in body cells. A woman experiences edema along with fatigue, headaches, and loss of strength. A potassium increase can bring the body back into sodium/fluid balance, which means that potassium may reduce a woman's bloatedness and, with that, headache, fatigue, and weakness may end. Potassium also aids muscle contraction and is important for normal cardiac function.

A woman may take potassium in liquid or tablets. Most prescribed potassium gluconate tablets contain 5 milli-equivalents (mEq.) of potassium gluconate. The recommended dose of two tablets four times daily, after meals and at bedtime, supplies 40 mEq. of potassium, the appropriate minimum daily requirement. The liquid dosage equals approximately 20 mEq. of potassium gluconate per tablespoon, and the minimum daily requirement is two tablespoons daily, or 40 mEq.

A patient with PMS might need two or three times the minimum daily requirement of potassium. This added dosage should not be a problem for a healthy individual, since a surplus of potassium is usually excreted without adverse reaction. However, a woman with renal or cardiovascular problems should not take potassium without checking with her doctor, because a high level of potassium can result in an irregular heartbeat and even death from heart failure if renal and cardiovascular conditions exist. Also, potassium can irritate the gastrointestinal system and, in some cases, cause ulcers and bleeding sores.

Potassium sold on the shelves in health food stores is available in either 83.5- or 99-milligram tablets. The milligram tablet dosage most likely equals 5 mEq. of potassium gluconate. A woman should be able to decipher dosage equivalents from the information on the potassium bottles.

A healthy PMS sufferer can increase her dosage from 8 to 20 tablets daily. However, she should be aware that these tablets can irritate the stomach and should be taken after, or in combination with, meals to avoid gastrointestinal upset. On the other hand, a new liquid potassium in a syrup base, which does not create gastrointestinal upset, may be the most advisable form of supplementation.

• **The B Vitamins.** As mentioned in Chapter 3, the "normal" American diet often lacks an adequate supply of the B vitamins, especially vitamin $B_6$, which is lost in cooking and canning, and when whole-grain breads or cereals are stored for a long time or exposed to light. Studies have shown that a vitamin B deficiency can affect the body's ability to regulate estrogen production. Without B vitamins, estrogen increases. Then an excess of estrogen causes a greater vitamin B deficiency and more estrogen is produced. It's a vicious cycle that leads to hormonal imbalance and PMS.

However, of all the B vitamins, a woman's greatest need may be for vitamin $B_6$ (also called *pyridoxine* or *pyridoxine hydrochloride)*, which appears to influence the release of the brain's neurotransmitters dopamine and serotonin. Neurotransmitters are mood regulators that may not be in adequate supply if a woman is deficient in vitamin $B_6$.

A vitamin $B_6$ deficiency may be inhibiting the production of dopamine and serotonin and causing a PMS sufferer to feel irrationally tense, depressed, irritable, or agitated. Vitamin $B_6$ supplements may stabilize such a woman's moods. PMS is a condition related to hormonal imbalance. Women who are on birth control pills are also in altered hormonal states, and studies have shown that many of these pill takers are subject to headaches, dizziness, fatigue, irritability, and depressions, which have been alleviated by vitamin $B_6$. It therefore seems logical that this vitamin, which brings relief in a time of hormonal change, would benefit a woman with PMS. Premenstrual food cravings and fluid retention may also subside with doses of vitamin $B_6$. However, it is important to remember that *vitamin $B_6$ should only be taken in combination with vitamin B-complex* to keep vitamin B intake properly balanced.

The B vitamins have been shown to influence the transmission of nerve signals that directly affect the release of the female hormones. To keep these neurotransmissions steady and accurate, every day a woman should take 100 milligrams of vitamin B-complex in combination with 50 to 200 milligrams of vitamin $B_6$. During the two weeks before her menstrual period a woman should increase her intake of vitamin $B_6$ to 500 to 800 milligrams daily. Since $B_6$ may cause stomach upset, it's a good idea to eat before taking this vitamin along with B-complex.

Vitamin B-complex with additional $B_6$ helps to alleviate the symptoms of PMT-D specifically, but these vitamins should really be considered a treatment for all forms of premenstrual syndrome. Even if a woman is being treated with progesterone or bromocriptine, which are described later on in this chapter, she should still continue supplementing her diet with the B vitamins. Medication increases the need for the B vitamins. There are many natural foods that are rich in the B vitamins. (See Table 1.)

• **Vitamin D.** Besides being found in fortified milk, tuna, liver, salmon, and cod liver oil, vitamin D is produced on the skin when a woman is in sunlight. People who spend most of their time indoors often do not have adequate supplies of vitamin D, which is very important in building calcium into the body.

## TABLE 1

## FOOD SOURCES RICH IN VITAMIN B

Liver and Brewer's Yeast (B.Y.) are the sources for the ten factors of the B Complex. Yogurt, buttermilk, kefir, acidophilus, and other cultured-milk products help encourage the growth of the Vitamin B–producing flora in the intestines.

| | |
|---|---|
| **B₁ Thiamine** | B.Y., soybeans, whole wheat (W.W.) bread, oatmeal, roasted peanuts, peas, pecans, walnuts, wheat germ, brown rice, lima beans |
| **B₂ Riboflavin** | B.Y., liver, kidney and heart, soybeans and flour, W.W. products, hickory nuts, hazel nuts, peanuts, turnip greens, mushrooms, peas, collards and kale |
| **B₃ Niacin** | Rice bran, rice polishings, roasted peanuts, liver, yeast, mushrooms, almonds, wheat, tuna, turkey, veal, chicken, peas |
| **B₆ Pyridoxine** | Bananas, avocados, green leafy vegetables, green peppers, cabbage, carrots, peanuts, B.Y., wheat germ, beef lever, W.W., halibut, molasses, oranges, sweet potatoes, raw pecans |
| **Biotin** | B.Y., liver, kidney, unpolished rice, soy flour and beans, eggs, cauliflower, roasted peanuts, mushrooms |
| **B₁₂ Cobalamine** | Difficult to obtain from natural sources |
| **Folic Acid** | Fresh, dark green leafy vegetables, liver, cauliflower, kidney and chicken giblets, lima beans, wheat germ, roasted peanuts, W.W., watermelon, asparagus, potatoes, cantaloupe |
| **Choline** | Egg yolks, milk, lecithin, oats, green beans, peanut butter, peas, spinach, wheat germ, soy beans |
| **Inositol** | Fruits and cereals, liver, B.Y., cantaloupe, grapefruit, oranges, peas, raisins, wheat germ |
| **PABA** | Yogurt, liver, yeast, wheat germ, blackstrap molasses |

Since vitamin D aids in the absorption of calcium, it should be taken in conjunction with calcium and magnesium supplements. A woman with PMS should consume 400 units of vitamin D three times a day to insure that the symptoms she is treating with calcium and magnesium have the best chance of being relieved. Without vitamin D, she may find that her symptoms persist.

• **Vitamin E.** There is some discrepancy of scientific opinion about the effectiveness of vitamin E, a nutrient naturally present in nuts, wheat germ, vegetable oils, and whole-grain breads and cereals. A Boston-based study concluded that women who took 400 or more units of vitamin E daily for two to three months showed improvement in their fibrocystic breast conditions. Other studies have not revealed vitamin E to aid in the healing of fibrocystic breast disease, but the research is still continuing. Meanwhile, perimenopausal and menopausal women seem to find relief from change-of-life symptoms with vitamin E. This vitamin prevents oxidation of fatty substances such as vitamin A, essential fatty acids, and the pituitary, adrenal, and sex hormones. To promote hormonal balance, a woman should take 400 to 800 units of vitamin E daily.

• **Vitamin A.** Dark green and orange vegetables such as spinach, broccoli, carrots, squash, sweet potatoes, and yams contain vitamin A, which originates from *carotene,* the yellow pigment in these foods. This vitamin is also in liver, butter, eggs, fortified milk, and margarine.

Vitamin A helps to maintain good vision, is necessary for the healthy development of bones and teeth, and aids fertility and lactation. Even more important, vitamin A fights infection by strengthening the immune system and helping the body attack disease, virus, and infection. Today, new studies are being conducted to learn the role that vitamin A might play in combating cancer. Since PMS can weaken a woman's resistance, especially if she is under stress while she has the syndrome, vitamin A may be particularly helpful to include in her vitamin regimen. A woman should take 5,000 units of vitamin A three times a day, in combination with her other vitamins.

• **Vitamin C.** Citrus fruits and juices are probably the most popular sources of vitamin C, which is also in pimentos, green peppers, strawberries, tomatoes, salad greens, and to a lesser extent in bananas, apples, and potatoes. Vitamin C builds and maintains *collagen,* the basis of the connective tissue that joins the body's cells and promotes healing. Vitamin C also fortifies the capillaries, builds iron into the bloodstream, and prevents other vitamins from being destroyed by oxygen. Studies are being done using vitamin C to block the development of nitrosamines, cancer-causing chemicals that enter digestive organs. With all this, vitamin C is a powerful weapon against illness.

When vitamin E is taken, vitamin C becomes depleted, so in order to maintain a good vitamin balance, a woman who is following a PMS mineral and vitamin plan should take at least 2,000 milligrams of vitamin C daily.

To reiterate, a woman should supplement her PMS nutritional diet with extra doses of the minerals calcium, magnesium, zinc, iron, and potassium, along with the B vitamins and vitamins D, E, A, and C. Each woman has to be her own detective, understand which minerals and vitamins pertain to her specific symptoms, and organize her personal supplementation plan. However, a woman may gain the most relief from her symptoms by taking every compatible mineral and vitamin in the regimen. Excessive minerals and vitamins, those consumed in doses that her body does not need, will in most cases be excreted.

• **Tryptophan.** As explained in the "Carbohydrates" section of the natural approach, the amino acid tryptophan is necessary to the manufacture of serotonin, one of the brain's mood regulators. It seems reasonable that if tryptophan is responsible for the creation of serotonin, and a low serotonin level can bring on depression, then a woman should be able to take tryptophan, increase her serotonin, and change the "blue" mood that may be part of her premenstrual syndrome. This appears to be a logical theory, but MIT researchers found that when volunteers who took tryptophan were psychologically tested, their feelings of joy or gloom were no different from those of volunteers on placebos.

Tryptophan may be increased by eating natural carbohydrates, as explained earlier, but many PMS sufferers, in spite of the MIT tests, continue to take tryptophan capsules with good results. In my practice, some patients say that they feel better on tryptophan, while others report no effects whatsoever. When a woman wants tryptophan, I suggest that she combine it with the nutritional plan described in this natural approach to PMS relief, and include vitamin B-complex in combination with additional vitamin $B_6$. As yet, there are no recommended B-vitamin dosages correlated with tryptophan's effectiveness.

A woman who is suffering PMS-induced depression might start on two 500-milligram capsules of tryptophan a day and increase her dosage to four daily capsules during her premenstruum. If she feels no effects from this dosage, she might take up to six capsules a day. Each woman, knowing her disposition and sensing her well-being, can judge better than anyone else what amount of tryptophan seems to improve her condition.

• **Evening Primrose Oil.** It has recently been discovered that the oil from the evening primrose flower is rich in linoleic acid, one of the body's essential fatty acids and the basis of prostaglandins. Hormonelike substances produced by the body's tissues, prostaglandins have at times been thought to influence premenstrual syndrome. However, there are many different kinds of pro-staglandins. The prostaglandins called PGE2 and PGF2 Alpha are the ones responsible for menstrual cramps, whereas PGE1 is the prostaglandin that is suspected of having a role in premenstrual syndrome.

A woman who takes an evening primrose capsule provides her body with linoleic acid for the increase of the PGE1 prostaglandin. (Linoleic acid is also naturally contained in vegetable oils such as cold-pressed safflower oil.) PGE1 lowers blood pressure, prevents blood clots, and may lower cholesterol levels and strengthen the immune system. It has been experimentally used as a treatment for alcoholism, eczema, schizophrenia, and as a hangover remedy. Not all of the claims for PGE1 have been proved but the research continues.

One of the reasons why evening primrose oil might help women with PMS is that it may influence symptoms that originate from the activity of the hormone prolactin. Dr. David Horrobin, a former professor of medicine at the University of Montreal, induced his own PMS symptoms when he injected himself with prolactin. The connection between prolactin and PMS has not been firmly established, though, and a relatively small number of PMS sufferers have high prolactin levels. Dr. Horrobin reports that symptoms may not depend on the amount of prolactin as much as on how the linoleic acid levels react with prolactin activity. The steady production of PGE1, which can be maintained with the linoleic acid of the evening primrose oil, may suppress PMS symptoms stemming from prolactin.

A British experiment with evening primrose oil was conducted by Dr. M. G. Brush at the Premenstrual Syndrome Clinic in St. Thomas's Hospital Medical School in London. Dr. Brush gave evening primrose oil to 65 PMS sufferers who had not been cured by other treatments, and at the end of his study 61 percent of the women had found total relief while 23 percent discovered that at least some of their symptoms had disappeared.

Dr. Brush's study is very encouraging and it shows, once again, that each woman's PMS is individualized. The treatment that works for one person may not be right for another. Evening primrose oil has been highly publicized. It is available at health food stores, but, at the cost of about twenty dollars for 100 capsules, which are only enough for two to three weeks, it is certainly an expensive treatment.

The first line of treatment for premenstrual syndrome should be a nutri-tional plan, mineral and vitamin supplementation, and stress reduction through exercise. If the natural approach is not completely effective, medica-tion might be necessary, but I would not suggest that a woman spend her money on evening primrose oil until she has tried other types of treatment.

## THE IMPORTANCE OF STRESS REDUCTION

When a woman is under stress, her premenstrual syndrome definitely intensifies. As mentioned in Chapter 3, the nervous system and the endocrine, or hormonal, network in the body make up the neuroendocrine system, which is the medical term that defines the complex and sensitive interplays between the brain's nerve signals and the body's fluctuating hormones.

Nerve-transmitting signals from within the brain affect the release of brain hormones from the hypothalamus and the pituitary, which in turn trigger hormonal action in other parts of the body. So although a woman's hormonal imbalance is responsible for the presence of PMS, this imbalance can be traced back to those initial chemical secretions in the brain, signals responding directly to stress. In fact, a high level of stress can inhibit the release of hormones to the point of making the syndrome unbearable.

Women who go through difficult times at work, or are faced with family problems, divorce, or coping with illnesses of loved ones, often find that their PMS symptoms deepen during these times. As a woman's stress increases, so does the severity of her symptoms. Then she may become even more emotionally depressed, less able to deal with stress, and her PMS symptoms may grow even more overwhelming.

A woman must step out of this vicious cycle by trying to reduce her stress through exercise and relaxation techniques. It is impossible to live in this world and never encounter stress, but a woman with PMS should know that she is especially susceptible to its effects. De-stressing techniques are important to her treatment program. In fact, all phases of the natural approach—diet, minerals and vitamins, exercise and relaxation—promote stress reduction. Even a woman's ability to share her knowledge of PMS with her friends and loved ones is a method of lessening inner tension.

If a woman allows herself to retreat from the world when she feels stress building, if she takes time for herself at home or at work, she will be striving to overcome her PMS. One television commentator married a man who had custody of his three children and suddenly found herself sharing a full house, when she had always lived alone. She felt incredibly pressured by new demands from four people at home until she finally seized on a way to reduce her stress. She took long, perfumed baths. Interestingly enough, no one questioned the time she spent in the bathroom. And alone in this stress-free environment, she was able to release her tension by soaking in the tub.

A woman with PMS needs stress-reducing habits. It is a good idea, for example, to avoid scheduling high-pressure meetings or emotional encounters when premenstrual syndrome is likely to be at its height. Of course, the best way of all for a woman to diminish stress and modulate the chemical secretions in her brain is through exercise. Physical activity releases the tension that stress has created. As oxygen enters the lungs, the heart pumps, the blood circulates, and the hormones flow.

Exercise is a significant part of the natural approach, but different kinds of physical exertion suit different people. Some women may prefer competitive sports such as tennis or racquetball, while other women may enjoy more solitary activities such as swimming, bicycling, or running. A brisk walk might be another good form of exercise. Two types of stress-reducing programs are presented here—daily exercises and yoga poses—so that a woman may choose the form she prefers. Even if a woman engages in sports, she will benefit from these at-home programs, which are specifically designed to help her conquer PMS. Both programs alleviate the physical symptoms of PMS while they reduce stress and improve psychological well-being. In addition, a meditation method is offered. Only ten minutes of meditation provides a woman with a sense of calm through a day of activity.

## METHODS OF STRESS REDUCTION

Moderate exercise tones the body, diffuses nervous energy, and lowers stress levels that often contribute to premenstrual problems. Women who are physically active usually have fewer complaints about PMS symptoms, since they are regulating the release of their brain chemicals and body hormones through exercise. They are also burning off fatty tissue, which, because it can be converted into estrogen, is a factor in estrogen/progesterone imbalance.

Aerobic exercises such as bicycling, jogging, or even strenuous walking are excellent ways of alleviating stress and diminishing PMS, but they should not be a woman's only source of stress reduction. It is important to stretch the spine, with its sensitive nerve endings, to strengthen the back and abdomen, and to send blood circulating through the reproductive organs if a woman is going to overcome PMS. A sufferer will find that the convenient at-home exercises described below in "The PMS Workout" and "Yoga Poses for PMS Relief" do all these things, while they are relieving stress.

A woman may choose either at-home exercise program, since both combine breathing and stretching techniques that reduce PMS as well as menstrual cramps. It is up to each sufferer to select the regimen that she finds is most compatible with her physical abilities. Also, as an important part of stress reduction, a woman might learn how to achieve an optimum state of relaxation by following the daily practice presented in the "Meditation" section.

## THE PMS WORKOUT

The personal fitness program provided by Olinda and Lazar Cedeno, founders of Exercise Plus in New York, offers an excellent method of stress reduction and PMS relief. A woman receives the greatest benefits from this workout if she does it every day. At the least, she should do it three times a week, and during her premenstruum she should increase the number of times to four or more. Olinda, her clients at Exercise Plus, and my patients have all reported relief from premenstrual and menstrual discomforts with these exercises. Situate yourself on a floor mat or on carpeting to begin. Here are Olinda's instructions:

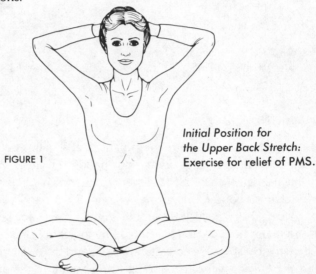

FIGURE 1

*Initial Position for the Upper Back Stretch: Exercise for relief of PMS.*

### Upper Back Stretch

Sit with your knees bent and legs crossed, Indian fashion. (See Figure 1.) Clasp both hands behind your head and point your elbows out to the sides. Keep your chest raised, shoulders relaxed, eyes forward. Open your mouth slightly and breathe in for two slow counts. As you breathe out, pull in your stomach as much as you can, round your back, and drop your chin to your chest. Close your elbows together. Drop your chin farther into your chest, pull in your stomach tighter, and stretch your upper back. Breathe in and rise up slowly to the original sitting position. Repeat the movement very slowly four times. On the fourth round, instead of returning to the original position, breathe in and out and begin stretching downward, aiming the top of your head toward the floor. Continue to round your back, pull in your stomach. Open your elbows. Breathe in and out with the downward stretch until your head practically touches the floor. (See Figure 2.) Relax your arms and hands on the floor. Breathe in and out and, with the head down, slowly roll up (See Figure 3), vertebra by vertebra, to a sitting position.

FIGURE 2                  FIGURE 3

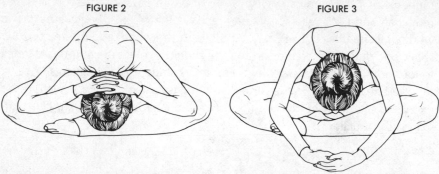

*Position 2 for the Upper Back Stretch: Exercise for relief of PMS.*      *Position 3 for the Upper Back Stretch: Exercise for relief of PMS.*

### Rhythmic Breathing

Lie on your back with your knees bent, feet slightly apart, and your arms on the floor alongside your body. Your hands and arms should be relaxed, with the palms of your hands either up or down, depending on what is comfortable for you. With your neck stretched out and your chin tucked in toward your chest, open your mouth slightly. Very slowly breathe through your mouth for two counts. As you breathe in, let the air fill first the abdomen and then the chest. Inhale on count one, expand the abdomen; on count two, fill the chest. Then slowly exhale, releasing the air in the opposite direction, first from the chest on count one, and then from the abdomen on count two. Press your entire spine against the floor as you breathe for eight slow, rhythmic rounds of inhalations and exhalations.

### Comfort Pose

In addition to diminishing PMS symptoms, this exercise offers relief from menstrual cramps any time during your period. Lie flat on your back. Bend both knees to your chest, relax your feet, and clasp each knee with a hand. Pull your knees down toward your armpits. Open your mouth slightly and breathe in for two counts, out for two counts. Breathe in and out for ten rounds, or as many times as necessary to relieve discomfort. Foot rotations increase circulation during the comfort pose. Point your toes, circle *outward,* and flex, five times. Point, circle *inward,* and flex, five times. (See Figure 4.)

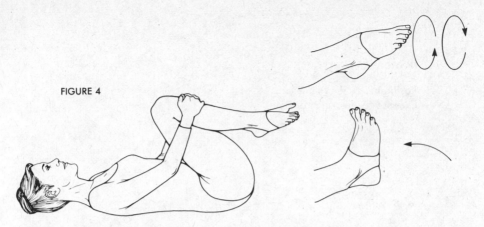

FIGURE 4

*The Comfort Pose for Relief of PMS:* Lie flat on your back with your knees pulled close to your chest. While in this position, point the toes of both feet and move each foot in a circular motion 5 times to the right (center drawing), flexing the foot with each rotation (bottom drawing). Follow these circular movements with 5 foot rotations to the left. Repeat these movements in cyclic fashion as many times as needed.

### Pendulum

Lie flat on your back. Bend your left leg and plant your left foot on the floor. Extend your right leg along the floor and flex your right foot. Relax your arms alongside your body. (See Figure 5.) Following the rhythmic breathing pattern, inhale for two counts. Slowly exhale for two counts, releasing the air, first from the chest, on count one, and then from the abdomen, on count two. As you breathe out, slowly elevate your right leg toward the ceiling. Keep the leg straight and the foot flexed as you lift your leg at a right angle to your body. (See Figure 6.) With your foot parallel to the ceiling, breathe in slowly for two counts. Breathe out for two counts and, as you are exhaling, pull in your stomach, tighten your buttocks, and begin to lower your leg toward the

FIGURE 5

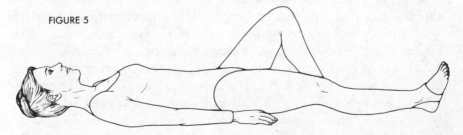

*Position 1 for the Pendulum.* Exercise for the relief of PMS.

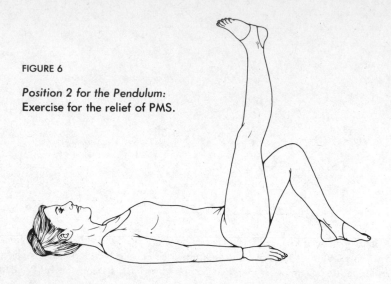

FIGURE 6

*Position 2 for the Pendulum:*
*Exercise for the relief of PMS.*

floor. Keep your knee straight, thigh tight, foot flexed, and squeeze the buttocks as you lower the leg, but *do not let your leg touch the floor.* Steady your leg an inch or two off the floor. Inhale for two counts, breathe out slowly for two counts, and once again, raise your right leg toward the ceiling and repeat the exercise. Complete six rounds of pendulum leg lifts, first with the right leg and then with the left leg.

### Forward Stretch

Sit in an upright position with your weight balanced on your buttocks. Extend your left leg along the floor and flex your left foot. Bend the right leg on the floor and place the bottom of the right foot against the side of the knee of the left leg. Raise both arms over your head, but make sure the arms are parallel to your ears. Reach your fingertips toward the ceiling. (See Figure 7.) Breathe in slowly for two counts. Breathe out and, while, exhaling, pull in your stomach, relax and slightly drop your head, round your back, and almost as if you are hinged at the hips, bend forward along the extended left leg. With your back rounded and your shoulders relaxed, try to reach for the toes of your left foot with your outstretched fingertips. (See Figure 8.) You do not have to touch your toes; in this exercise the stretch is important. Breathe in, breathe out, and while exhaling, raise back to the seated upright position with your hands and arms overhead. Breathe in slowly for two counts, breathe out and repeat the forward stretch for a total of six times along the left leg. Then reverse leg positions and repeat the exercise six times along the right leg.

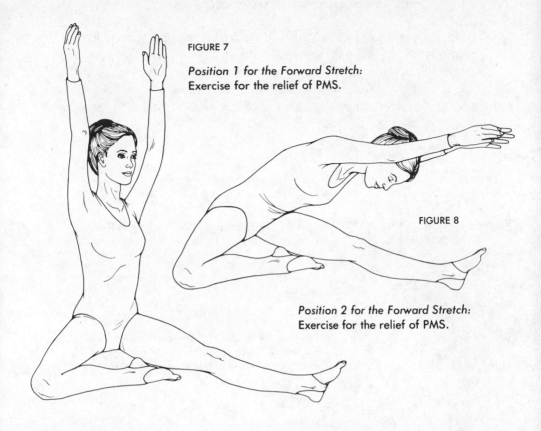

**FIGURE 7**

*Position 1 for the Forward Stretch:*
*Exercise for the relief of PMS.*

**FIGURE 8**

*Position 2 for the Forward Stretch:*
*Exercise for the relief of PMS.*

## *Relaxation*

Stand with your feet spread at a distance about the width of your hips. Raise your arms parallel to your ears, fingertips reaching toward the ceiling. (See Figure 9.) Breathe in slowly for two counts, breathe out for two counts, and while exhaling, pull in your stomach and slightly bend your knees. Keeping your arms aligned with your ears, drop your arms and head, then your upper torso, toward the floor. Round your back as you descend, and lower your hands as far as you can down to the floor. (See Figure 10.) Grasp the backs of your ankles with your hands, and while you are in this inverted position, breathe in for two counts. Breathe out for two counts, and while exhaling, pull in the stomach and stretch your head between your legs. (See Figure 11.) Relax, breathe in for two counts, breathe out, and once again, while you are exhaling, pull in your stomach and stretch your head between your legs. Repeat the breathing and stretching for a total of four rounds. After the fourth round, release the ankles, let the arms hang loosely, straighten the legs, and allow your upper body to dangle. Breathe in for two counts and

**143**

balance your weight on the balls of your feet. Breathe out, pull in your stomach, and slowly roll the spine, vertebra by vertebra, up to a standing position. Your arms are at your sides. Head is high and face is forward. This is the end of the relaxation exercise, in which the blood has flowed in an opposite direction, circulation has increased, and the back and spine have been stretched and relaxed.

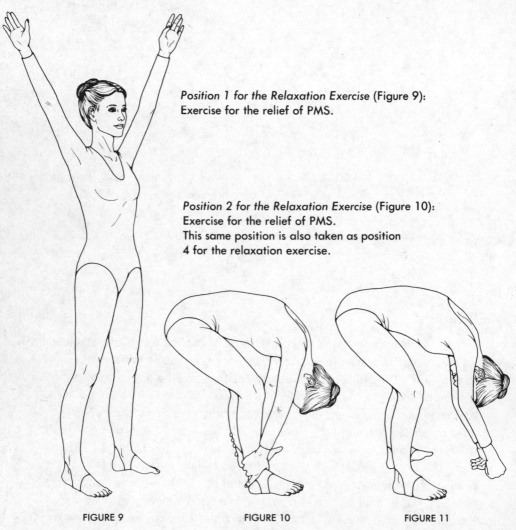

*Position 1 for the Relaxation Exercise* (Figure 9):
Exercise for the relief of PMS.

*Position 2 for the Relaxation Exercise* (Figure 10):
Exercise for the relief of PMS.
This same position is also taken as position
4 for the relaxation exercise.

FIGURE 9          FIGURE 10          FIGURE 11

*Position 3 for the Relaxation Exercise* (Figure 11):
Exercise for the relief of PMS.

## YOGA POSES FOR PMS RELIEF

Yoga is an ancient Eastern discipline through which a person gains control of the mind and the body, and aims to achieve inner tranquility. The exercises that are part of the yoga discipline lift the stressful pressures that afflict the mind and, at the same time, relax and strengthen the body. Dr. Loren Fishman, who specializes in physical medicine and rehabilitation at Albert Einstein College of Medicine in New York, is also an experienced yoga instructor. He spent three years in India studying and mastering the discipline, and for many years since, he has privately conducted yoga classes.

Dr. Fishman has discovered that certain yoga poses have helped to alleviate the discomfort of premenstrual and menstrual problems experienced by his female students. He has provided instructions for these poses, which should be done on a floor mat or carpeting. Ideally, a woman should perform these poses every day, but if her scheduling does not permit a daily exercise routine, a yoga program at least three times a week will still help to diminish her PMS symptoms within three months. She will feel the benefits of yoga by holding each pose for as long as she can up to one minute.

Yoga exercises are not individually repeated the way the exercises are in the PMS Workout; instead, yoga exercises are, as mentioned before, *poses* that a woman maintains. As she becomes more accomplished in the yoga technique, a woman will find that she can hold the poses more easily, but at the start, she may only be able to remain in a pose for thirty seconds or less. Without straining, as she continues the program, she should work toward becoming more flexible and extending her time in each pose.

Dr. Fishman has included the ancient Sanskrit names for the yoga poses along with his instructions. He advises women to do the poses in the following sequence:

### The Palms-to-Heaven Pose (Parvattanāsana)

Sit on the floor with your weight balanced on your buttocks. Your body should be symmetrical. Shoulders are positioned parallel to your hips. Bend the left leg at an approximate 60-degree angle. As you bend the right leg, place the outside of the right foot on the left thigh. Position the foot as close to the groin as possible but do not strain. When the right foot is resting on the left thigh, the right knee should be able to lean on the arch of the left foot. It is important that you are in a comfortable cross-legged position, so place the right foot only as high on the left thigh as your flexibility permits. (See Figure 12.) If you are inflexible and cannot touch your right foot to the left thigh, you may sit in an Indian-style cross-legged position, but you should work to achieve the proper yoga pose to attain the benefits of the exercise.

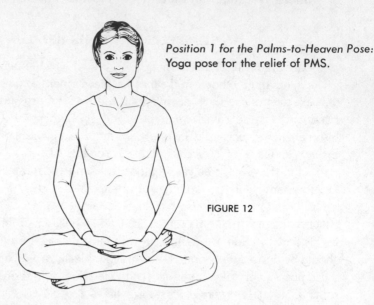

*Position 1 for the Palms-to-Heaven Pose:* Yoga pose for the relief of PMS.

FIGURE 12

Let your hands form a basket in your lap by placing your left hand in the palm of your right hand. At this point, the head and shoulders are evenly supported by the spine. Bring the hands about a foot in front of your navel. Interlock the fingers. Thumbs remain free. Inhale for two counts, exhale, and begin to elevate your hands. When your hands reach face level, inhale and slowly turn your hands, palms outward, raising them toward the ceiling. Extend the elbows, straighten the arms over your head, and exhale. The palms of your interlocked hands are facing the ceiling. (See Figure 13.) Press your arms toward each other behind your ears. Bring your shoulder blades together and stretch from the lower back, up the arms to the fingers. Breathe evenly through the nostrils. With each inhalation, stretch even higher toward the ceiling, and at the same time relax the sphincter muscles.

Hold this balanced, palms-to-heaven pose for thirty seconds, or as long as your can. The spine is slightly arched, and the arms are extended. After you have held the pose as long as possible up to one minute, relax the shoulders, relax the elbows, and slowly release the grip of the hands. Return the hands to your lap in an easy, circular motion. Inhale. Exhale. Reverse the leg positions. Bend the right leg at an approximate 60-degree angle. Bend the left leg and place the outside of the left foot on the right thigh. Repeat the pose in the reverse leg position.

This pose strengthens the abdominal wall, stretches uterine and ovarian ligaments, and increases the circulation around the reproductive organs. Also, the upper body stiffness which often accompanies PMS is significantly reduced or entirely eliminated.

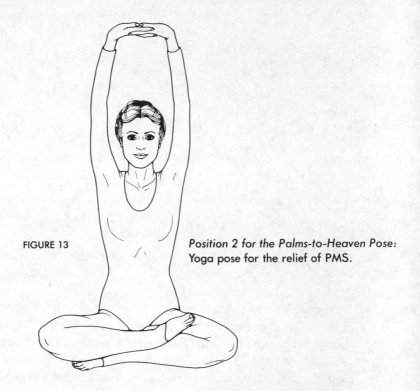

FIGURE 13

*Position 2 for the Palms-to-Heaven Pose: Yoga pose for the relief of PMS.*

### Toner for the Internal Organs (Baddha Konāsana)

*Part 1:* Sit on the floor with your weight balanced on your buttocks. Legs are outstretched with the feet flexed and about three feet apart. Place the hands palms down on the knees and arch the back slightly. Inhale deeply. Exhale slowly and, during the exhalation, aim the head and eyes toward the ceiling, remove the palms from the knees, and place the hands on the floor. Crawl forward with the fingertips. The upper body is straight but inclining forward, as if it were hinged at the hips. Little by little, the fingers crawl forward and the entire torso lowers toward the floor. The eyes continue to seek a high point on the ceiling. (See Figure 14.) When the exhalation is complete, stop, rest, and inhale. Exhale and crawl foward again. When you have crawled as far as possible with your fingertips, hold the pose for as many seconds as you can up to one minute. Keep the eyes fixed on the ceiling, the back slightly arched. Breathe slowly and evenly through the nostrils. When you have held the pose as long as possible, relax the hands and slowly drag them backward along the floor as you return your body to an upright seated position. Bend the knees and comfortably bring the legs together.

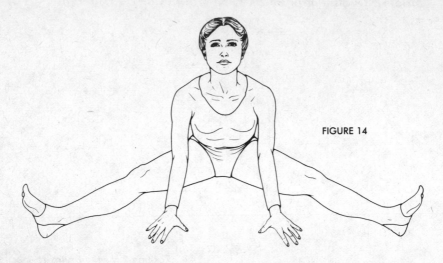

FIGURE 14

*Position for Part 1 of the Toner for the Internal Organs:* Yoga pose for the relief of PMS.

*Part 2:* After completing Part One, while sitting in the balanced, upright position, bend the legs with knees outward, and bring the soles of the feet together. The bottoms of the feet are facing and touching each other. Firmly grasp the feet with the hands and bring the heels as close to the the body as possible. (See Figure 15.) The feet should not leave the floor and the sides of the legs and knees should be as close as possible to the floor. If the knees are

*Position for Part 2 of the Toner for the Internal Organs:* Yoga pose for the relief of PMS.

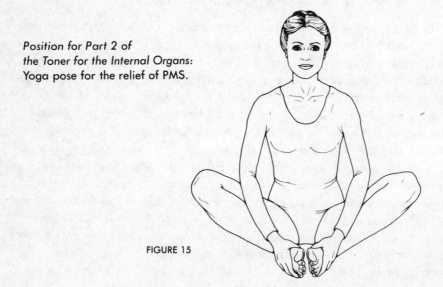

FIGURE 15

not even near the floor, release the hands and press the elbows into the creases of the bent knees. Gradually allow the knees to descend toward the floor. If the knees are still far away from the floor, position yourself against a wall in the Part Two pose. Touch the lower spine, pelvis, back, and head to the wall and continue pressing the knees toward the floor. Contact with the wall helps to lower the knees.

When the knees are as close to the floor as possible, the bottoms of the feet are touching, and the hands are pulling the feet in toward the body, hold the pose as long as possible up to one minute. The back is straight, the shoulders are back, and the eyes are looking directly ahead. This is a difficult pose and you may find that you are only able to hold the position for ten seconds. In time you will be able to remain in the pose longer. When you are finished holding the pose, release the hands and slowly straighten the legs. This pose stimulates the ovaries, helps to regulate the menstrual cycle, and even aids in childbirth.

### Pelvic Twist (Marichyāsana)

Sit on the floor with the legs extended and the feet flexed. With the hands pressed on the floor directly beside the hips, balance the weight on the buttocks. Bend the right leg and position the right foot high up against the inside of the left thigh. The right hand is placed on the floor at a point close to the body behind the buttocks. The right arm is fully extended and straight. The right shoulder is turned toward the right hand.

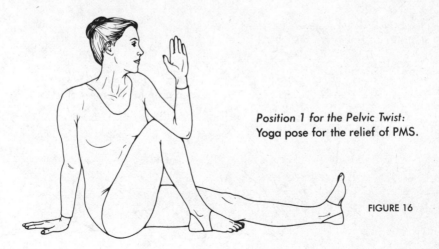

*Position 1 for the Pelvic Twist:
Yoga pose for the relief of PMS.*

FIGURE 16

Raise the left arm so that the elbow clears the top of the right knee and passes to the outside of the right leg. Ease the left shoulder beyond the right knee by turning the torso from a point just above the waist. Raise the left forearm so that it is in an exact vertical position. The hand is open, fingers pointing up. Turn your face directly forward, gaze straight ahead. (See Figure 16.) Press the left upper arm against the outside of the right knee. The left elbow extends just a little beyond the right knee. Maintain the twist by pressing the left arm against the right leg while pointing the right shoulder toward the right hand. The shoulders should be turned to a point where they are almost parallel with the left leg. Keep the body weight balanced as much as possible. Maintain body symmetry and do not allow the weight to shift to the left buttock. To intensify the twist you may want to move the right hand a little farther behind you. To twist even more, some women may want to lower the left arm and grasp the left leg with the left hand. Hold the pose for at least thirty seconds. Work up to one minute if possible.

To release the pose, grasp the right thigh with the left hand. (See Figure 17.) Slowly return the right hand to the front of the body from its extreme posterior position. As the right hand comes around, release the left arm from its pressure on the right thigh. Slowly slide the left arm and hand up the thigh and over the right knee. You are relieving the pressure that the twist has put on the spine. Place both hands on the floor beside the hips. Then with the hands pressed on the floor directly beside the hips, balance the weight on the buttocks. Keep the right leg extended with the right foot flexed. Bend the left leg and position the left foot next to the left knee. Repeat the pose in the reverse leg position.

FIGURE 17

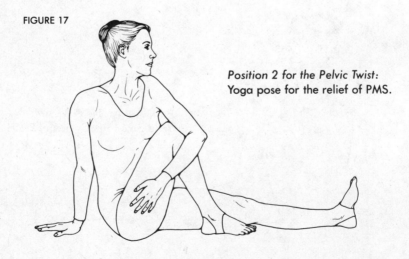

*Position 2 for the Pelvic Twist:*
**Yoga pose for the relief of PMS.**

The pelvic twist gives great flexibility to the spine and massages the internal organs with a gentle but pervasive pressure. The kidneys, adrenal glands, and female organs are especially affected by the internal massage. Hormonal imbalances and abdominal muscular aches can be relieved by this pose.

### Minimal Inverted Pose (Beginning of the Jathara Parivartanāsana)

Sit on the floor with your right side against the wall. Your body is parallel to the wall. Place the left hand at a right angle to your side and slide your left hand and arm along the floor until you are resting on your forearm and left elbow. Turn your upper body toward the left arm and place the right hand on the floor to support yourself as you lower your body and slide your left arm along the floor until it is fully extended. You are now lying on your left side flat on the floor. The buttocks are touching the wall. Bend the knees.

The head is resting on the extended left arm. Keeping the left arm straight, lower it from the shoulder until it is parallel to the wall. Pressing the weight on the right hand and left arm, turn onto your back by pivoting on the left hip. Extend the legs against the wall. The buttocks should be directly against the wall. Flex the feet and stretch the legs as far as possible. (See Figure 18.) The backs of the thighs, knees, calves, and heels should lean directly against the wall. Hands and arms are extended alongside the body. Lower the shoulders and bring the shoulder blades flat against the floor.

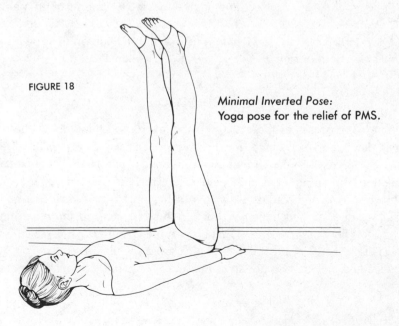

FIGURE 18

*Minimal Inverted Pose:*
**Yoga pose for the relief of PMS.**

Slide the fingers along the floor until the knuckles are actually touching the wall. Stretch the back of your neck and tuck the chin in toward the chest. Relax the stomach muscles and lower the small of the back to the floor. Try to touch the entire spine to the floor. Relax the face and eyes. Inhale slowly and symmetrically through the nostrils. Fill the body with air. Exhale slowly, releasing the air first from the chest and lungs, and then from the abdomen. Remain in this pose as long as you can up to one minute.

To come out of the pose, bend the knees to the chest. Raise the right arm out from the shoulder until it is at a right angle to the body and parallel to the wall. Turn onto your right side by pivoting on your right hip. For support, place the left hand on the floor above the right arm. Draw the right arm out from underneath the body. Place both hands on the floor and assume a crawling position on your hands and knees. Sit back on your legs. This pose, like all the other yoga poses, should be done once every day, or at least three times a week.

Even in this minimal inverted pose, the blood supply to the kidneys is somewhat reduced. This temporary change in circulation stimulates urination, making the pose a natural diuretic that can reduce bloatedness. On the other hand, although the kidneys may receive less blood, the heart and lungs have a greater blood supply. The inverted pose also sends additional blood to the head, stimulating the thyroid, pituitary, and pineal glands, and massaging the brain membrane, which, when it swells, influences the severity of the migraines, irritability, tension, and depression, the symptoms of premenstrual syndrome.

Dr. Fishman recommends that for further information on therapeutic yoga poses women turn to the writings of B. K. S. Iyengar.*

## MEDITATION

Everyone possesses the ability to meditate. If you think about the way a child daydreams, sometimes much to a parent's chagrin, you will realize that the youngster is only temporarily retreating from reality to maintain a balanced state of mind. A child who is constantly stimulated by new people, objects, colors, and sounds allows her or his mind to be "at rest" for a time. This is not a learned behavior, but a natural reaction to the environment. Thoughts flow purposelessly. Then, when the child returns to reality, she or he is "refreshed" and ready to deal with more stimuli.

As adults we often do not allow our thoughts to drift off unless it is the end

*B. K. S. Iyengar, *Light on Yoga* (New York: Schocken, 1966).

of the day and we are just about to fall asleep. We are regularly assaulted by problems from which we do not mentally escape. Then the body reacts physically. Tension, frustration, and anxiety build to the point of affecting hormonal fluctuations. When a woman has PMS, her symptoms intensify with stress.

However, every woman can regain the talent for mental refreshment that she had as a child. She can rediscover a technique that permits her to deal with stress before stress debilitates her. Women find that they are better able to maintain good mental health and to cope with stressful stimuli when they meditate every day. What a child does without "thinking" a woman must learn to do, but once she starts to include ten minutes of meditation in her daily routine, she will notice that her tolerance for coping with stressful events increases. And as stress becomes less bothersome, there is a good chance that PMS symptoms will noticeably diminish.

Ron Shapiro, a stress management consultant who is in private practice in New York, advises his clients to set aside ten minutes each day for meditation. Every woman who is trying to overcome the symptoms of PMS might benefit from stress reduction through meditation by following Mr. Shapiro's instructions:

• ***Schedule a ten-minute period that is free from interruption.*** Select a time of day when you are relatively free from demands. Many people find that the early hours offer quiet, contemplative periods, but you must choose the part of the day that best suits your routine. Then, once you choose a time to be alone for ten minutes, stick to it with determination. If you've carefully scheduled your time, it will not conflict with your responsibilities to others, and the members of your household will respect your privacy. Have a timer, set for ten minutes, close at hand. Do not answer telephone calls during your ten minutes alone and make sure that everyone close to you understands that you want to be by yourself.

• ***Choose a place that you can go to every day.*** You will be sitting in a straight-backed chair that you should put in a private area away from activity. If you cannot find an out-of-the-way spot, locate yourself where activity can flow around you without including you. You should face toward something visually uninteresting. Since you are trying to avoid distractions, do not decorate this place. Let the spot remain impersonal, but know that it is always there. It is important to meditate at the same time, in the same place, every day.

• ***A total stretch-to-the-limit.*** Before sitting down to meditate, lift your arms overhead, reach toward the ceiling, and stretch your body to its limit. You will feel a pleasant resistance and a tingling warmth will follow. Now you are ready to assume the sitting position.

• *A comfortable sitting position.* Use a firmly constructed, preferably straight-backed, chair that allows you to sit in a comfortably erect position without need of a back support. You may want to place a small cushion at the curve of your buttocks to give you a slight forward tilt. Keep both feet slightly apart on the floor. Balance your weight evenly on your buttocks and sit in a relaxed posture with your hands placed palms down on your knees. Lower your head slightly; a raised chin promotes an aggressive attitude, and you are aiming for a kindly demeanor. Keep your eyes open, mouth closed. Breathe through your nose.

• *Set aside animosity.* Once you are comfortably seated, speak inwardly to yourself about your determination to suspend angry thoughts for ten minutes. You are not going to dwell on animosity you may feel toward yourself and others. Compose a sentence that you inwardly repeat. For example, the sentence may be: "For these ten minutes, I will set aside my anger at the world and at myself." Hear the statement being spoken in your own inner "voice."

• *The three-breath visualization.* Now imagine a natural scene of great beauty, perhaps a place where you have been. One woman who has traveled in Africa imagines a fiery red, orange, and gold sunset on the veldt. Giraffe and zebra are silhouetted against the sky. As you visualize your personal scene, whether it is a mountain vista or ocean waves breaking at the shore, breathe in deeply and slowly. Breathe out quietly and softly, slowly releasing the air from your lungs. Complete a total of three deep inhalations and exhalations and permit the scene to fade. Now breathe quietly. Make no effort to regulate your breath, just allow it to continue at its own rate.

• *Alert, attentive sitting.* You will become aware that your thoughts are less active. They are quieting down. Continue to sit comfortably erect and try not to move. Remain silently attentive. Feel the stillness and resist any urge to shift position, scratch, or sniff. Do not make any noise. Breathe through the nose. Your mouth is closed. Now focus your attention on distant sounds that make themselves heard. Do not feel that you have to identify or explain them, just listen dispassionately. Let the sounds be like a kind of background music that you hear but do not judge. Continue to sit this way until the timer rings. (An alternative to "listening" during "alert, attentive sitting" is called "counting your breaths." Rather than focusing your attention on distant sounds, concentrate on counting your inhalations and exhalations. Breathe in, count one; breathe out, count two—until you count to ten. Then begin another round. Every time you reach ten, start from one again. Count your breaths until the timer rings.) Do not stand immediately. Hesitate for a moment. After a short pause, as you rise up, sense your posture. Are you comfortably erect?

Balanced? Are you still attentive? Consciously attempt to carry your awareness into your day's activities.

There is no reason for a woman to test her endurance and see if she can meditate longer than ten minutes when she begins the practice. Although the time period may be extended, it is best to become accustomed to the ten-minute interval before increasing it. After a few months, if a woman is firmly committed to the practice of meditation, she may want to change her time to twenty minutes. She may even consider membership in a small group in which her meditation technique may be refined by an experienced teacher.

## SLEEP

Women who suffer from PMS often have hormonal imbalances and hormonal levels that make them more fatigued. A woman should not feel embarrassed to admit that she may need more sleep during her premenstruum than she does at other times of the month. In fact, she should probably get at least eight hours of sleep a night, so that she will be better able to manage stress and lessen her susceptibility to anxiety and nervousness.

If a woman's sleep patterns have been interrupted by symptoms of premenstrual syndrome, then she should avoid caffeine-containing beverages and chocolate and choose a method of stress reduction, either the PMS Workout or yoga, in addition to practicing meditation. These stress-relievers make the mind and body relaxed and ready for sleep.

Sometimes warm milk with honey can help a woman to fall asleep. A small snack before bedtime can also be conducive to sleep because it relaxes the stomach; although food might provide a short spurt of energy, it will soon result in a hypoglycemic episode that brings on fatigue and overcomes insomnia.

Pharmaceutical sleep aids are discussed in "The Medical Approach to PMS Relief"; however, most PMS sufferers are very sensitive to drugs and should avoid sleeping pills. Using the natural approach, two to three 500-milligram tablets of tryptophan in the evening may help to stabilize a woman's mood swings and bring on a sleep-filled night.

The natural approach, which includes a nutritional program, mineral and vitamin supplementation, and methods of stress reduction, is the first line of treatment for PMS. A woman may plan her own natural approach after she identifies her PMS symptoms. Each woman's mineral and vitamin requirement is different, and although it is often best for each woman to put together her own supplementation program, there is one vitamin supplement that is especially designed to help women with perimenopausal and premenstrual symptoms. This multivitamin-mineral supplement, called Optivite, has been formulated by Dr. Guy E. Abraham. Vitamin C, B₆, magnesium, and zinc are the main components of Optivite. This vitamin supplement reportedly relieves premenstrual tension, irritability, breast engorgement, bloatedness, sweet cravings, and lethargy, and reduces difficulty in coping with stress. Optivite should be available in local health food stores, but if a woman cannot find it, she can write to the manufacturer, Optimox, Inc., Rolling Hills Estates, California 90274.

If the natural approach does not completely curb a woman's symptoms, she should arrange to visit a doctor who treats premenstrual syndrome, or a PMS clinic, for an examination, counseling, and hormonal analyses through blood tests. It is possible that she might have a severe hormonal imbalance that has not been corrected with the natural approach. It is also possible that other gynecological problems that affect the severity of her PMS may exist. Each case of premenstrual syndrome is unique and a woman owes it to her good health to get sound advice and proper care. Treatment through the medical approach, which includes prescription medications in addition to the natural approach, may be needed; however, medications should never be considered "the cure." Drug therapy can only enhance the natural steps that a woman is taking toward recovery.

## *The Medical Approach to PMS Relief*

A woman needs a doctor or a PMS counselor with good judgment and a thorough understanding of the complexities of premenstrual syndrome to suggest the appropriate treatment. If the natural approach has not successfully diminished her symptoms, or if the results of her blood tests show hormonal imbalance, a sufferer becomes a likely candidate for prescribed medication.

However, gauging the dosage and the course of the treatment is a tricky matter. Hormonal fluctuations vary from month to month and they respond to changes in daily life. Stress and travel, for example, affect hormonal secretions and alter the need for PMS medication. Therapy that was beneficial one month may become inadequate another month, or on the other hand, the necessity for medication may disappear entirely. A new hormonal imbalance may require a stronger dosage of a prescribed medication, or a sudden hormonal *balance* may make medication superfluous.

A PMS sufferer is sensitive to the ups and downs of her body, and she will probably know before her doctor does whether her medication is making a difference. She is likely to recognize her biological need for a change of dosage or a suspension of treatment. A woman and her doctor must work together over the course of several menstrual cycles to find the proper therapy, and the best way for a woman to join in the treatment process is from an informed position.

It is important for a PMS sufferer to understand the dosage and the effects of the hormonal supplementation or other medications that her doctor may recommend, and she must also be alert to "wrong" advice. If a doctor suggests a hysterectomy, a D&C, tranquilizers, antidepressants, or pregnancy to cure her premenstrual syndrome, she should find another physician. In fact, it is a good idea for a woman to know what she should *not* do, even before she begins to educate herself about the medical treatments that are effective against PMS.

## WARNING: BEWARE OF INAPPROPRIATE CARE

Time after time I have heard women describe years of living on antidepressants and tranquilizers because they were diagnosed as psychotics. These women were later proved to be PMS sufferers, and they eventually became physically and emotionally stable. They had only to be taken off antidepressants and tranquilizers, and properly treated with a combination of the natural and medical approaches to feel "normal." For years, lives that could have been happy were tragic. However, in comparison with other sufferers, these patients were lucky. The mistakes that were made on them were at least reversible.

Some women have submitted to hysterectomies that were advised by physicians who felt that removal of their organs was the only way to eliminate their problems. Of course, what followed in many cases was immediate surgical menopause, which brought on hormonal difficulties that were often more pronounced than PMS symptoms.

If a woman who believes she has PMS visits a doctor who suggests any of the treatments listed below, she should decline to accept his advice and make an appointment with a different physician. The treatments that are inappropriate to combating PMS, and may even cause more serious health problems, are:

• *Hysterectomy*. As recently as a few months ago, I received letters from women who described hysterectomies they had agreed to for PMS relief. A majority of them were told that all their troubles resided in ovaries that were not producing correct amounts of estrogen and progesterone. The operation given on many occasions was a *total hysterectomy with a bilateral salpingo-*

*oophorectomy,* which entails removal of a woman's uterus, ovaries, and tubes.

Removal of the organs does not cure PMS, and this surgery, as with all surgeries, puts a woman at risk of complications from anesthesia and unforeseen events during the procedure. Also, when the ovaries are excised, a woman no longer produces estrogen and the disappearance of this female hormone can lead to calcium depletion, bone weakening, and osteoporosis, as well as debilitating menopausal symptoms. A woman can experience hot flashes, severe mood swings, depression, weight gain, and a loss of her sex drive. A doctor may then try to help her overcome these problems with synthetic hormones, which may have a detrimental effect on her health in the long term, and might possibly cause cancer.

If a woman is suffering uncontrollable bleeding or she has been diagnosed as having cancer, a hysterectomy might be necessary to save her life. However, if PMS is her problem, she should "run as fast as she can" from the doctor who suggests hysterectomy as the cure.

• *Dilatation and Curettage (D&C).* During a D&C the cervical canal is dilated—opened with metal rods of increasing diameters—and a curette, an instrument with a sharp-edged open loop, is used to scrape excessive tissue from the uterine cavity. For years, patients believed that a D&C could cure all ailments. However, only heavy bleeding caused by uterine polyps or excessive uterine tissue can be cured by a D&C, and most certainly PMS, which results from hormonal imbalance, will not be helped by this surgery. In fact, there is no surgery that is effective in treating PMS. Even a laparoscopy, which gives a doctor a chance to "take a look" at your organs, will not help. The hormonal imbalance in your body cannot be corrected through surgery; therefore, if surgery is suggested, seek a second opinion.

• *Tranquilizers.* Many physicians have treated PMS symptoms with tranquilizers such as Valium. It is perhaps even possible that the popularity and subsequent abuse of Valium was partly caused by misdiagnosis of PMS. Doctors mistakenly attributed the symptoms of depression, irritability, panic, mood swings, crying, as well as headaches and migraines, to stress and nervousness easily overcome with a few Valiums. Many women who later learned of their premenstrual syndromes reported that their symptoms had intensified when they were on tranquilizers. This is common. When women have PMS, their depressions deepen with tranquilizers.

A woman must not accept tranquilizers as a principal line of treatment for her PMS, but if she is exceptionally anxious, she might be prescribed a mild tranquilizer on a limited basis. In this instance, the tranquilizer is an adjunct to her treatment program. A new European tranquilizer called Xanax (talprazolam), easy to remember because it is spelled the same front to back and vice versa, is now available in .25- and .5-milligram tablets that may be taken two or three times a day. With Xanax, a woman may lessen her anxiety without subjecting herself to long-lasting, depressive effects. Remember, though, that even the mildest of tranquilizers should only be taken in rare instances when anxiety cannot be controlled by any other means.

• *Antidepressants*. If a woman's strongest complaint is depression, with accompanying irritability and agitation, she may encounter a doctor who attempts to relieve her symptoms with an antidepressant. An antidepressant drug has to build in potency within the body and it takes some time before a woman feels any effect from it. Since a PMS depression is a cyclic one that is not always present, it seems illogical to suggest treatment with an antidepressant. A woman who has a serious PMS-induced depression should carefully follow the suggestions given in the sections "The B Vitamins" and "Tryptophan," which are part of the natural approach.

If after having been counseled by a knowledgeable physician or PMS specialist, and having tried a combination of the natural and medical approaches, a woman is still despondent, she should, only as a last resort, allow a mild antidepressant into her treatment program. An antidepressant such as Elavil (amitriptyline) or Tofranil (imipramine hydrochloride), 25 milligrams three times a day for a limited period, may be helpful. Also, Limbitrol (chlordiazepoxide, 10 milligrams and amitriptyline, 25 milligrams in one tablet), one tablet three times a day, might occasionally be indicated. Never, though, should the use of an antidepressant be suggested as the first or best way to help a woman overcome premenstrual syndrome.

• *Pregnancy*. Obviously, PMS, a condition created by hormonal imbalance during the course of the monthly cycle, will not appear when there is no cycle, when menstruation is arrested as it is during pregnancy. Hormonal levels are steady—estrogen and progesterone are in balance during childbearing—and a woman does not experience PMS. But the creation of another human being is hardly a way to overcome premenstrual problems. And what happens after pregnancy? Women have reported that PMS symptoms become even more severe, and it must also be remembered that many women who were not previously sufferers have been known to experience the syndrome after childbirth. If a doctor advises pregnancy purely as a means of overcoming PMS, a woman should leave his office and not look back.

## WHAT A DOCTOR SHOULD DO

When a woman consults with a doctor to have her suspicions of PMS confirmed, she should expect a physical examination, as described in Chapter 4. The battery of blood tests that are also explained in Chapter 4 will be ordered by the doctor if he feels her case warrants further investigation.

When the time comes for the doctor to suggest medication based on his findings, a woman should ask to see her records. It is her right to study and understand every hormonal analysis that has been conducted, and her doctor should willingly clarify the details of her case. He may feel she has other types of menstrual distress in addition to PMS, and he may want to treat these conditions while he is formulating his medical approach.

A woman should have a complete understanding of any medication that she is advised to take. An antiprostaglandin will calm menstrual cramps and Danocrine combats endometriosis, but neither medication is specifically aimed at conquering PMS, although they might occasionally be used as supplementary treatment. On the other hand, medications such as Synthroid, Parlodel (bromocriptine), progesterone, and spironolactone, which directly affect hormonal activity, are possible sources of PMS relief. All of these prescribed medications, and more, are detailed in this chapter.

## THE ROLE OF ANTIPROSTAGLANDINS IN THE TREATMENT OF PMS

As explained in the "PMS vs. Menstrual Cramps" section of Chapter 4, a woman may suffer premenstrual syndrome along with menstrual cramps. However, while PMS results from a hormonal imbalance, scientists have recently found that menstrual cramps are caused by high levels of prostaglandins, hormonelike substances that may be significantly present in the lining of the uterus as well as in other body tissues.

If a woman who has symptoms of PMS mentions menstrual cramps as one of her discomforts, and her doctor rules out abdominal pain from infection or tumors or other kinds of pelvic disease, her cramps are probably being caused by prostaglandins. In this case, the doctor may decide to treat her with an antiprostaglandin, a medication that inhibits the release of prostaglandins and thus alleviates cramps.

An antiprostaglandin is an aspirinlike medication, and in fact, before she takes a prescription drug, a woman who has not tried aspirin for her cramps might take two aspirins four times a day for two days *before* her period starts, and during the first days of her flow. A woman must be especially sensitive to her menstrual cycle in order to time her antiprostaglandin medication accurately.

If aspirin seems ineffective, Midol, which is a specific menstrual-pain reliever, should be the next remedy considered since it also inhibits the release of prostaglandins. Midol should be taken correctly, however. The recommended regime is two Midol tablets, four times a day, two days *before* and during the first few days of menstruation. This regimen has freed many women from the agonizing grip of menstrual cramps.

A doctor might include aspirin or Midol in his suggested medical approach to PMS relief, or he might favor a prescribed antiprostaglandin medication. Three prescription drugs recently approved by the FDA for relief of menstrual cramps—Motrin (ibuprofen), Anaprox (naproxen sodium), and Ponstel (mefenamic acid)—are often more effective than aspirin in blocking prostaglandins. In fact, prescription antiprostaglandins have been so welcomed by women that the list of these drugs is growing. Feldene (piroxicam) and Dolobid (diflunisal) might someday also be available. Since the inhibition of prostaglandins reduces the pain and swelling caused by arthritis, these medications, on the market as arthritis-pain relievers, are being studied for use in the relief of menstrual cramps.

One to two tablets of either Motrin, in 400-milligram tablets, or Anaprox, in 275-milligram tablets, taken four times the day before menstruation and continued during the first few days of bleeding, curb cramps and lessen the menstrual flow. Motrin is also now available in 600-milligram tablets, and one tablet taken four times the day before menstruation and during the early days of a woman's menstrual period is another alternative. Also, a woman may take one 250-milligram Ponstel tablet four times daily, starting the day before menstruation and into the first few days of her flow.

Of the drugs under study, Feldene is available in 10- and 20-milligram doses taken twice a day, and Dolobid is recommended in an initial 1,000-milligram dose, followed by 500 milligrams every twelve hours. Since all antiprostaglandin medications can irritate the stomach and gastrointestinal tract, they should be taken with some food, a piece of cheese or a cracker.

Once again, it is important for a woman to remember that her doctor is prescribing antiprostaglandins for her menstrual cramps, not for her PMS. Motrin or Anaprox, for example, will only supplement her overall PMS treatment. Her premenstrual syndrome requires a combined natural, and possibly medical, approach for her complete recovery.

Some PMS sufferers complain of pelvic cramping and tension headaches, which occasionally can be alleviated with antiprostaglandins—such as Midol, Motrin, or Anaprox—taken one to four times daily during the premenstrual days, when the symptoms are most severe.

## WHY A DOCTOR MAY PRESCRIBE DANOCRINE IN THE TREATMENT OF PMS

Endometriosis, which is described in detail in the "PMS vs. Endometriosis" section of Chapter 4, is a disease in which the tissue that forms the endometrium, the lining of the uterus, spreads to the organs outside the womb. When a healthy woman menstruates, the vascular endometrium sloughs off and leaves the body as menstrual blood. However, a woman who has endometriosis retains fragments of the vascular tissue within her abdomen. This leftover endometrial tissue then responds to the hormonal fluctuations of the menstrual cycle. Stimulated by the female hormones, it grows and spreads.

Endometriosis, like premenstrual syndrome and menstrual cramps, is a form of menstrual distress. The symptoms of the disease include a possible painful ovulation two weeks before menstruation, severe cramps during menstruation, and a deep abdominal pain on one side or the other, or an unspecific abdominal pain before or after menstruation. Other signs are infertility and pain during sexual intercourse.

When a woman describes these symptoms to her doctor, in addition to those symptoms created by PMS, he may begin to suspect endometriosis. He may even discover endometrial growths when he examines a woman internally. Endometriosis may exist alone, in combination with premenstrual syndrome, or in association with menstrual cramps and PMS.

Danocrine (danazol), a synthetic antihormone, is the only medication that is FDA-approved for treatment of pelvic endometriosis and fibrocystic breast disease (FBD). Danocrine blocks the release of the brain hormones FSH and LH, which stimulate a woman's ovaries to release a monthly egg. Therefore, Danocrine prevents ovulation, and without ovulation, there is no endometrial buildup, no menstrual flow, and no chance for endometriosis to spread. Danocrine also blocks hormonal receptors in the endometrial tissue. While a woman is on Danocrine, her estrogen and progesterone remain on the same steady low levels that are normally found after menstruation, a time when most women feel their best.

If a doctor finds that a woman has endometriosis, he may advise her to take Danocrine—200-milligram tablets two, three, or four times daily depending on her symptoms—for six to nine months. During this time the endometrial tissue will start to disintegrate and slowly be reabsorbed by the body until it disappears entirely.

While it is *the medication* for endometriosis, Danocrine is not normally used as a treatment for PMS. However, I have in my practice found that many PMS sufferers whom I have treated for endometriosis have said that their premenstrual syndrome disappeared along with their disease. Apparently, since Danocrine steadies hormonal fluctuation for several months, the body has a chance to hormonally readjust itself. In many instances, a complete remission of PMS occurs after a course of Danocrine.

A woman who is suffering with endometriosis and premenstrual syndrome should certainly be treated with Danocrine. Also, a woman who is suffering from fibrocystic breast disease, either alone or in combination with PMS, is a candidate for danazol treatment. Since Danocrine steadies a woman's hormonal levels, it could be tried as a treatment for PMS in cases where other approaches have failed.

## WHAT TO EXPECT FROM THE MEDICAL APPROACH

A number of medications that affect hormonal activities are being given to today's PMS sufferers. Treatment with progesterone has probably received more attention than other medications, but not every woman needs progesterone.

For example, PMS relief may come from regulating the thyroid gland, or from inhibiting the production of the brain hormone prolactin, or by influencing the flow of the adrenal hormones. A doctor can administer medications that perform each of these tasks.

As I have often repeated, every sufferer's syndrome is unique. If a woman's case shows that she needs more than the natural approach, she can augment her recovery plan with medication that she and her physician or PMS consultant agree is right for her. However, it may take several menstrual cycles to arrive at the dosage that conquers her condition. A woman's patience and determination, more than anything else, will lead to her victory over PMS.

## THYROID MEDICATION IN THE TREATMENT OF PMS

Hormonal secretions from the thyroid gland stimulate the brain's releasing hormones, which in turn trigger hormonal activity in the ovaries. In some women, this chain reaction may make the thyroid responsible for an estrogen/progesterone imbalance that brings on PMS.

When depression, agitation, frustration (generally the symptoms of PMT–D) are highly noticeable during a woman's premenstruum, she might have a malfunctioning thyroid gland causing her syndrome. After noting her symptoms, a doctor should order the T3 and T4 thyroid tests, as described in Chapter 4, for analysis of the hormonal activity of her thyroid.

The results of the T3 and T4 tests might vary from laboratory to laboratory, so a doctor should carefully scrutinize all lab reports. If he sees a low, or what is called a "low-normal," reading for thyroid function, he should prescribe a minimal dose of thyroid medication. If a woman's reading is exactly in the middle of the "normal" range, her thyroid function is probably all right, but anything less than a precise "normal" may be the source of her PMS depression. I have seen numerous women overcome their depressive symptoms after a course of thyroid medication. In fact, studies have shown that one out of seven women hospitalized for depression recovered after their thyroid conditions were treated.

A doctor might suggest a thyroid medication such as Synthroid (levothyroxine sodium), 50 to 100 micrograms daily, for PMS relief. This thyroid medication should be taken for months, and possibly years. After a year's time, a woman might be tested to see if the treatment is still necessary.

A woman should be alert to any changes she feels while she is on thyroid medication. A dosage that is too high may cause nervousness and insomnia. A dosage that is too low may have no effect on her symptoms. In general, the proper dosage of thyroid medication for a woman who has below-normal function increases her metabolism, gives her energy, and alleviates her depression.

Besides Synthroid, other available thyroid medications that appear to be especially helpful in the treatment of PMS are Cytomel (liothyronine sodium) and Armour Thyroid tablets prepared from dessicated animal thyroid glands.

## PROLACTIN SUPPRESSION IN THE TREATMENT OF PMS

The pituitary gland in the brain is the source of prolactin, a hormone that stimulates the secretion of breast milk. In most healthy women, prolactin does not vary much during menstrual cycles, but at times, the body's prolactin flow can be linked to a woman's emotional responses. If a woman is under any kind of psychological stress, her prolactin level may rise. This hormone has been known to increase in response to suction on the breast, pain, frustration, upcoming surgery, and sexual intercourse. Studies have also shown that the hormone reaches high levels at various times throughout the menstrual cycles of women who have premenstrual syndrome.

A high prolactin level may signal the presence of small tumors, called *microadenomas,* in the pituitary gland, and a woman should be checked for this condition.

It is important to know that as prolactin rises, different symptoms appear. A slightly increased prolactin level may bring on PMS by inhibiting the fluctuations of the brain hormones FSH and LH, which affect the production of the female hormones estrogen and progesterone. A moderately high prolactin level has even greater impact on hormonal production and may result in shortened menstrual cycles, heavy menstrual flows, and PMS symptoms such as edema and weight gain, which are related to an excess of estrogen. Eventually, an especially high prolactin level can cause *amenorrhea,* a disappearance of the menstrual flow, and a condition called *galactorrhea,* which is a leakage of breast milk from the nipples.

When prolactin levels are high, a drug called Parlodel (bromocriptine mesylate), which blocks the production of this hormone, stops milk secretion if it exists, and reinstates the synchronized fluctuation of the brain and the female hormones. Studies have shown that when treated with bromocriptine, 30 percent of PMS sufferers with high prolactin levels find relief. However, quite curiously, 30 percent of the sufferers with normal prolactin levels are also helped.

Studies of the effectiveness of Parlodel (bromocriptine) in combating PMS are not yet conclusive. In a recent double-blind study in which one group of women were treated with bromocriptine and another group received place-bos, both groups found relief from PMS symptoms. Many of my own patients with high prolactin levels have reported improvement with the drug, but it does not help in every case.

Parlodel seems most beneficial to women who have symptoms such as fluid retention and breast tenderness. For example, if a woman who is on progesterone therapy is especially bothered by painful breasts, she may be given Parlodel along with her progesterone treatments. Sometimes a doctor may suggest Parlodel to a patient whose prolactin level has not yet been reported by the lab that is analyzing her blood tests. The reasoning is that if 30 percent of women who have normal prolactin levels feel better on bromocrip-tine, why not try it if everything else fails. However, since prolactin levels can be determined through blood tests, a woman might prefer to ask her doctor to wait until the results of her tests are in before she agrees to this medication.

Parlodel causes a number of side effects. Nausea appears in 50 percent of the patients who take it. To much lesser degrees, headache, dizziness, fatigue, abdominal cramps, constipation, and diarrhea have also been reported. When a woman is being treated with Parlodel, to minimize its side effects, she should at the start take a low dose of the medication with her evening meal. Parlodel is available in 2.5-milligram tablets. She should take a half tablet with dinner for several days, beginning two days before the expected onset of her PMS symptoms. Dosage may be increased to one whole tablet in the evening if she has not felt relief with the half-tablet dosage. A second tablet may be taken with breakfast if a woman still has not experienced improvement and if she has no side effects. Some women find relief from PMS with low doses of Parlodel—a half tablet two or three times a day—but many sufferers need a 2.5-milligram tablet two or three times a day to overcome their syndromes. A severely afflicted sufferer should take bromocriptine, two to three tablets daily, starting on the tenth day of her cycle and continuing until menstruation.

## PROGESTERONE TREATMENT FOR PMS

A carefully orchestrated fluctuation of the female hormones estrogen and progesterone occurs during the menstrual cycle. As explained in Chapter 3, progesterone markedly increases after ovulation, when it is abundantly produced by the corpus luteum, the ovarian scar tissue that remains after the newly ovulated egg begins its journey through the Fallopian tube. This is the second half of the menstrual cycle, the luteal phase.

The progesterone that is being naturally secreted by the corpus luteum passes to the endometrium, the uterine lining, in increasing amounts from the time of ovulation to menstruation. Progesterone levels usually peak in the last week of the cycle and sharply drop a day or two before menstruation. The rise in progesterone, which characteristically occurs at some point during days 21 to 23 of the cycle, often coincides with the time that women with progesterone deficiencies notice symptoms of PMS. By the way, if a woman conceives, her progesterone will not drop, as it normally does before menstruation. Progesterone is the hormone that maintains pregnancy. During the first two months of expectant motherhood, progesterone is secreted from the ovary in escalating amounts. After the first two months, and until the end of pregnancy, progesterone is secreted by the placenta.

A hormonal imbalance between estrogen and progesterone has been found in PMS sufferers who complain of symptoms that show they have the PMT–A type of syndrome, as explained in Chapter 2. Anxiety, irritability, nervous tension, hostility, and depression are part of PMT–A.

A woman who exhibits PMT–A may successfully overcome her symptoms with the natural approach. Modification of her diet, mineral and vitamin supplementation, and stress reduction may alleviate her syndrome. However, if her case of PMS is extremely severe, and she finds no relief through the natural approach, then she may be helped by progesterone supplementation. As explained in Chapter 4, a blood test taken at a point in the menstrual cycle when symptoms are pronounced can reveal the ratio of progesterone to estrogen. A doctor may even take blood tests during more than one cycle to confirm his readings. He should be interested in specifying the ratio between progesterone and estrogen, not in judging how close each hormonal level comes to what a laboratory considers "normal" values.

There is one problem with blood tests, however. Although researchers can determine hormonal levels in the bloodstream, they cannot identify hormonal levels in body tissue. Progesterone and estrogen receptors exist in tissues, and these receptors affect the way the body responds to hormonal levels. A woman's blood test may not show an imbalance of the female hormones, but her clinical symptoms may indicate that such an imbalance exists. This discrepancy may be due to the fact that the receptors present in body tissue may be causing the imbalance.

A doctor may base his treatment on his evaluation of a woman's clinical symptoms, whether or not he can scientifically verify an imbalance. He may decide to administer progesterone on the grounds that he feels such hormonal supplementation is a sound medical approach. Fortunately, only a minority of women who suffer from PMS will need progesterone treatment. If an imbalance does show up on a blood test, it may be that the progesterone is lower than normal in the luteal phase of the menstrual cycle. Sometimes a progesterone deficiency may have been interpreted as an excess of estrogen before the blood test. This happens because the more potent estrogen level, which is caused by the low progesterone, is creating symptoms of an estrogen excess, fluid retention and weight gain for example, which are strongly felt by the body.

Progesterone is usually the treatment of choice for a woman with a hormonal imbalance caused by too little progesterone and too much estrogen. Progesterone is also indicated for women who are suffering from PMS symptoms severe enough to interfere with their daily routines. When marital and family lives are affected and the safety of children is at stake, progesterone should be administered. Progesterone is also suggested if there are signs that PMS may lead to suicide attempts, self-injury, increased alcohol consumption, or cyclic illness that requires hospitalization. Torturous, recurring migraines that cannot be curbed with other medications may provide another reason for progesterone therapy.

If progesterone is deemed necessary, a woman may only need treatment for a few cycles to regulate her hormonal fluctuation. It is possible the body will be able to readjust itself so that progesterone can be slowly decreased and eventually eliminated. As explained in the "How Progesterone Is Administered" section in this chapter, this hormone cannot be taken in oral capsule or pill. Progesterone is administered through suppository, injection, or implantation, methods that are less convenient than swallowing liquids or pills. But the use of progesterone, which is also expensive, may not have to last for long. PMS sufferers have been able to balance their hormonal fluctuations after just a few months on progesterone. Women taking this mediction must still continue the natural approach, with reduced salt intake, frequent small meals, avoidance of refined carbohydrates, and high doses of vitamin B-complex and vitamin $B_6$.

## HOW PROGESTERONE TREATMENT EVOLVED

Years ago in England, Dr. Katharina Dalton noticed that her own menstrual migraines disappeared during the last six months of her pregnancy. Conferring with another physician, Dr. Dalton concluded that the high levels of progesterone present during pregnancy might have made the difference. She decided to test her theory personally, and in the dual roles of doctor and patient, she injected herself with progesterone every day. Just as she had suspected, her menstrual migraines vanished. Dr. Dalton then tested the use of progesterone on other women. When she was called in to care for a woman who was hospitalized for severe asthmatic attacks, the woman's husband told her that his wife had a seizure every month except when she was pregnant. Dr. Dalton was able to cure the woman with progesterone, and what would become her well-known advocacy of this now international treatment took hold. Since then, many other physicians throughout the world have followed her example and have successfully treated PMS sufferers with progesterone.

## DIFFERENCES BETWEEN NATURAL PROGESTERONE AND SYNTHETIC PROGESTOGENS

When a doctor suggests progesterone treatment, a woman should make sure that he is talking about giving her *natural progesterone* and not synthetic progesterones, called *progestogens* (or *progestagens*). *Only natural progesterone is effective in combating premenstrual syndrome.* Progestogens do not diminish PMS and may even worsen a woman's symptoms, although a couple of my patients have found relief on synthetic progestogens (Provera).

Researchers wanted to create a synthetic form of progesterone because natural progesterone was very expensive to produce. Furthermore, natural progesterone could not be taken in pill form, since it is not absorbed into the bloodstream as an oral medication. A natural progesterone pill disintegrates in the stomach and gastrointestinal tract and never enters a woman's system. Synthetic progestogens were designed to simplify any treatment that called for progesterone, and the differences between progestogens and natural progesterone were never especially significant to doctors. Most physicians believed that one could replace the other. Although natural progesterone and synthetic progestogens are interchangeable in many instances, the treatment of PMS is not one of them.

Natural progesterone, a cholesterol derivative, is made from Mexican yams, soybean products, and, occasionally, from animal sources. Progestogens are chemically formulated from progesterone, but rather than duplicating the properties of progesterone, these synthetic hormones react differently.

In addition to exhibiting the progesterone effect, some have estrogenic effects, some have *very potent* progesteronelike effects, and some also react like male hormones. Birth control pills contain the synthetic progestogens, which is why women with PMS may feel debilitated when they're on the pill.

Both a synthetic progestogen, such as Provera, and natural progesterone can trigger uterine bleeding similar to a menstrual flow. However, one of the problems with the synthetic progestogens is that they inhibit a woman's natural progesterone production. Synthetic progestogens actually lower the concentration of natural progesterone in the blood and, in fact, worsen the imbalance of the female hormones and intensify the symptoms of PMS. Some progestogens are actually 2,000 times more potent than progesterone, which is why certain progestogens can make women feel more out of sorts than others.

Also, the synthetic progestogens that have testosterone activity—such as norethynodral, ethisterone, dimesthisterone, and norethisterone—can have masculinizing effects on a woman, while the synthetic progestogens with estrogen activity bring on symptoms such as fluid retention and edema, which are related to an estrogen excess. Natural progesterone, on the other hand, does not cause masculinization and is known to *reduce* sodium and fluid retention.

Synthetic progestogens, in addition, are unable to function as progesterone substitutes in an essential biological conversion process that involves progesterone and the adrenal glands. In the body, natural progesterone is converted into hormones called *corticosteroids* by the adrenal glands. These corticosteroids aid in transporting *glucocorticoids* through the bloodstream. Glucocorticoids regulate the body's blood sugar metabolism. If progesterone is low and the adrenal conversion does not occur, a woman may experience a drop in blood sugar that brings on a hypoglycemiclike episode. If she is taking synthetic progestogens, they may be responsible for this episode because, first, progestogens do not convert into corticosteroids and, second, they serve to lower progesterone levels. This temporary hypoglycemia may be corrected with progesterone supplementation, however.

Both natural progesterone and synthetic progestogens may be helpful in maintaining pregnancy, although synthetic progestogens should not be used since they might harm fetal development. This adverse effect on the fetus has not been reported when natural progesterone has been used during pregnancy. In fact, studies of the offspring of women who took natural progesterone during their pregnancies have revealed that these children are especially intelligent and well-adjusted. Among the adverse effects that have been observed when certain progestogens have been taken during pregnancy is that the sex organs of female babies have become somewhat masculinized.

Progesterone is not believed to be cancer causing. No human cancer has been reported during progesterone treatment; quite the reverse, progesterone has been used in treating specific uterine cancers. One animal study, however, found that synthetic progestogen injections caused breast cancer in beagle dogs. The synthetic progestogens involved in this study have been removed from the market!

As mentioned earlier, when a woman is treated with synthetic progestogens, her body becomes confused and produces less natural progesterone. When natural progesterone drops, the hormonal conversion by the adrenal glands cannot take place, salt may build up, fluid may be retained, and hypoglycemia may ensue. Synthetic progestogens generally make PMS symptoms worse, so if a woman is about to be treated with progesterone, she should be sure that it is *natural progesterone*.

## WHY HASN'T THE FDA APPROVED PROGESTERONE FOR PMS?

Until women began to learn about premenstrual syndrome and recognize their need for treatment, the demand for progesterone suppositories in the United States was low. Basically, suppositories were available in 25- to 50-milligram doses that were usually prescribed to correct luteal-phase deficiencies, often in women who were being treated for infertility due to repeated miscarriages. Before the recognition of PMS, there were few conditions that required a progesterone cure.

In England, however, Dr. Dalton and her colleagues have been treating women with 400-milligram progesterone suppositories for years. The higher-dose suppositories are manufactured under the name Cyclogest by L. D. Collins & Company in Hertfordshire, England. These suppositories cannot be exported to the United States, though, since the required FDA double-blind testing of progesterone has not yet been performed. L. D. Collins is a small British company that is not equipped to conduct the elaborate and expensive tests required by the FDA. It has been estimated that to market a new drug—which is what high-dose progesterone is now being considered—can cost as much as $74 million.

FDA spokespeople have said that they are worried about possible serious side effects from high doses of progesterone, and the agency is withholding its approval until these high doses can be tested. The fact that for more than a decade Dr. Dalton has been treating women with 400 or more milligrams of progesterone a day, and that her patients have experienced no serious side effects, is apparently considered irrelevant by the FDA. The agency has set a 200-milligram per day limit on progesterone used in testing. So far, there have been no conclusive findings, but most patients who require progesterone seem to need a somewhat higher dose.

Right now, natural progesterone is being compounded by individual pharmacists who are responding to requests from physicians treating PMS. Major drug companies, which are usually eager to conduct studies and compete for the patent on a new drug, have been reluctant to establish testing programs that may lead to FDA approval of progesterone. One of the main reasons for hesitation in the industry is that the patent on the natural extraction of progesterone ran out decades ago. Therefore, a company could spend millions of dollars on research and not have rights to the product they have tested. Remember, progesterone is natural and a company cannot patent something that is supplied by nature.

A company might be able to patent a *method* of releasing progesterone into the body, a timed-release capsule or suppository perhaps, but at the moment, no pharmaceutical firm has committed itself to progesterone research. And even when the FDA studies begin to bring results, the fact that a 200-milligram ceiling has been set for testing ultimately may not prove helpful. Of the minority of sufferers who require progesterone, some women need higher doses, because vaginal and rectal absorption differs from one woman to another.

There are even occasions when women do not respond to progesterone treatment. In a 1976 paper, "The Menstrual Cycle and Mood Disturbances," written by Dr. S. L. Smith and published in *The Journal of Clinical Obstetrics and Gynecology,* Dr. Smith did not report any significant effects from treating a number of patients with depressive symptoms with progesterone. The women in the study were given alternate-day injections of 100 milligrams of progesterone from day 19 to 26 of their cycles. Progesterone is not expected to be effective in cases of PMS in which severe depression is the main symptom. Even Dr. Dalton has reported that progesterone is not effective in all cases. On the other hand, in several papers she has explained how women have been successfully and continuously treated with progesterone without suffering serious side effects. Since Dr. Dalton has cared for thousands of PMS sufferers, her findings should be respected. (Note: Some side effects may result from progesterone treatment, and these are discussed later on in this chapter.)

The present research needs careful scrutiny. Psychiatrist Gwyneth A. Sampson's often-quoted paper, "Premenstrual Syndrome: A Double-Blind Controlled Trial of Progesterone and Placebo," published in the *British Journal of Psychiatry* in 1979, states that women overcame symptoms of PMS whether they were on progesterone or placebos. However, several of the women who were selected as PMS sufferers for her study were suffering from menstrual distress (symptoms such as menstrual cramps), and not premenstrual syndrome. Progesterone is ineffective in the treatment of menstrual cramps. Since all the patients in Dr. Sampson's study did not appear to be PMS sufferers as defined in this book, her findings, according to my interpretation, are inconclusive. Thus, it is wise for a woman to remain skeptical and read between the lines of any publicized reports about the effectiveness of progesterone.

I have seen hundreds of women whose lives have dramatically changed after they have been carefully counseled, examined, and treated with the natural approach in combination with two or three menstrual cycles on progesterone. A former PMS sufferer, and a patient of mine, recently described her recovery from PMS with the following words, which almost sound like an advertisement for progesterone: "I never thought I had the capability to run my own life, to do something outside the house, but now I'm in charge of my own business. I have self-confidence and self-esteem and I owe it all to progesterone." This woman was once rushed to the hospital to be treated for attempted suicide. Other women could be quoted, but the point would be the same, over and over: PMS is real and progesterone helps to cure it if a hormonal imbalance is found. Soon the government will not be able to deny that fact. With hope, the FDA will soon alter its chauvinistic approach to women's health care and begin to realize the importance of treating the total person. The FDA at present is ignoring the need for medication that can correct an imbalance of the female hormones, which is solely a woman's problem. It is amazing that the government appears to be more concerned with the effects of natural progesterone than they are with the well-known side effects of tranquilizers (such as suicide and addiction). New tranquilizers are regularly approved by the FDA.

## HOW PROGESTERONE IS ADMINISTERED

A woman should only begin progesterone treatment when her blood tests or symptoms indicate that it is necessary. As mentioned earlier, progesterone in pill form is destroyed in the stomach and gastrointestinal tract before it has a chance to enter the bloodstream and change the body's hormonal balance. Since oral medication does not work, natural progesterone is usually administered by either vaginal or rectal suppositories, or through intramuscular injections. (Dr. Katharina Dalton has also treated PMS by implanting compressed pellets of pure progesterone into abdominal fat, but her implantation method is not widely used.)

Progesterone is most commonly administered by suppository. A woman who is prone to vaginal infection or cystitis should be advised to use rectal medication, whereas vaginal suppositories are recommended for a woman who has few vaginal difficulties, or for a woman with excretory problems. With the suppository method, progesterone slowly builds in the bloodstream. Intramuscular injection creates a rapid rise of progesterone in the blood, and the hormone is slowly excreted. In twenty-four to forty-eight hours a woman needs another injection.

Progesterone suppositories slowly melt in the vagina or rectum. As a suppository dissolves, the hormone is steadily absorbed by the mucous membranes and, finally, enters the bloodstream. This little-by-little increase is more easily tolerated by the body than the sudden hormonal surge brought on by injection. However, the rate of absorption varies from woman to woman. It is felt that only 25 to 50 percent of the prescribed dose of progesterone ever reaches the bloodstream and becomes effective. Since there is such a range in the absorption capability of each person, a doctor and a patient must work together over the course of several menstrual cycles to find a woman's optimum dosage.

The FDA recommends that progesterone treatment begin with 25 milligrams twice daily in suppositories. If a woman is not relieved, her dosage may be increased, but it should not exceed 100 milligrams twice daily. Dr. Dalton feels that progesterone dosage is gauged by whether or not a woman has borne a child. For a woman who has never given birth, Dr. Dalton recommends 200 to 400 milligrams of progesterone in vaginal or rectal suppositories, or 50 milligrams in a daily intramuscular injection. Women who have borne children are advised to take 400 milligrams twice daily in suppository form, or 100 milligrams through intramuscular injection. Dr. Dalton also suggests that women increase their dosages up to three or four times the recommended amounts if they are not experiencing relief. Women who continue to suffer under treatment might have poor absorption, according to Dr. Dalton.

I have prescribed progesterone treatment when it seems that all other avenues of recovery have been unsuccessful. At the point when progesterone is needed, I have found that 25 milligrams is generally insufficient for relief. The lowest effective dosage in my experience is 50 milligrams of progesterone in suppository form, twice daily. This dosage may be increased three or four times daily, if a woman does not feel better on the lower amounts. Most of my patients need up to 200 milligrams twice daily, and sometimes women require 200 milligrams three or four times daily, if their symptoms continue unabated. However, I usually do not recommend that a woman take over 800 milligrams a day. On occasion I have suggested a higher dosage, but only for a short time.

• **When to Begin the Treatment.** A woman should begin combating her PMS with progesterone two days before the expected onset of her symptoms. PMS sufferers usually notice symptoms two to fourteen days before their menstrual flows begin, but of course the timing of each woman's symptoms is different. If a woman's syndrome starts fourteen days before menstruation, she is experiencing PMS at ovulation and the condition is continuing until her period. It is important for a woman to calculate her cycle and determine the arrival of her symptoms, in order to know when she should begin medication. Treatment starts two days before her symptoms are due.

Usually, thirty minutes after a suppository is inserted, progesterone begins to enter the bloodstream. If a woman is taking the appropriate dosage of progesterone, her symptoms will not appear. She should continue to use the suppositories until her period is due. For example, if she expects her period on Tuesday, she should stop her treatment on Monday night.

Most women on progesterone treatment take the medication from ten to fourteen days a month, stopping at menstruation and starting two days before the anticipated onset of PMS. However, some women have extremely severe symptoms while they are menstruating. These sufferers are advised to halve their doses and use rectal suppositories during the first few days that they flow. Once again, it is worth repeating that each woman's syndrome is uniquely her own. Her strength of dosage and duration of treatment must be specially formulated. A woman and her physician must join together as partners in her health care.

Once she finds relief with a specific dosage of progesterone, a woman should continue that dose for three or four additional cycles. Then she should gradually reduce or stop her dosage.

• **Where to Obtain Progesterone**. If a woman is being cared for by a physician who routinely treats premenstrual syndrome, or by a counselor at a PMS clinic, either of them may be able to supply her with progesterone that has been previously ordered by prescription. She may also find that she can purchase suppositories inexpensively by bringing her prescription to a local pharmacist who can custom-produce a suppository from progesterone powder in a combination Carbowax base PEG 400 and PEG 8000.

Also, a number of pharmacies across the country will fill individual prescriptions sent by doctors who are treating PMS. One of these pharmacies is Madison Pharmacy Associates, 1603 Monroe Street, P.O. Box 9641, Madison, Wisconsin 53715. Madison Pharmacy will fill a prescription for injectable progesterone and suppositories, in whatever dosage is requested by a physician. Progesterone in a rectal suspension, which has been specially formulated by Madison Pharmacy, is also available by prescription. This liquid progesterone formula is administered with a small syringe. Leakage is less likely with the rectal suspension, which enters the bloodstream faster than suppositories and is half their cost. Madison Pharmacy's gelatin capsule filled with progesterone is available as an alternative to the wax-based suppository. While some women might prefer the capsule, it is not as efficient a treatment as the suppository method. Suppositories that are sold in prescribed quantities usually cost about a dollar apiece, but prices vary according to the progesterone dosage of the suppositories, and the charges set by the pharmacy producing them. Bulk manufacture of progesterone suppositories awaits FDA approval.

## SIDE EFFECTS OF PROGESTERONE TREATMENT

Physicians who treat PMS and counselors at PMS clinics have been quoted as saying that there are "no side effects" from progesterone. But PMS sufferers have said something different. Women on progesterone treatments have reported that they were experiencing side effects, that there were a number of discomforts connected to the use of progesterone. They have mentioned leakage from the suppository, a change in sex drive, and an assortment of other things.

What the doctors probably meant by "no side effects" was that no *serious* side effects such as cancer, diabetes, hypertension, or other major problems had been observed. Dr. Dalton has repeatedly reported that there is no risk of cancer from progesterone. This hormone is actually used in fighting cancer— uterine cancer and some vaginal cancer that appears in young women whose mothers took diethylstilbestrol (DES) during their pregnancies.

Dr. Dalton probably has more experience with PMS treatment than any other doctor in the world. For years she has treated women with doses of 400 milligrams twice daily, sometimes three times a day, and one would expect that with these relatively high doses some major side effect would have emerged by now. Also, Great Britain, where Dr. Dalton practices, is the country that discovered the major side effects of the birth control pill. British medical professionals are constantly on the alert for side effects from drugs, and they are not likely to accept a medication unless they are satisfied that it is safe.

In the United States, thus far, the FDA reports that animal studies show that high doses of progesterone for long periods may change the body's metabolism and lipid count, but there have been no studies to determine whether high doses of progesterone could cause cancer.

The confusion about progesterone and cancer stems from studies in which synthetic progestogens injected into beagle dogs caused breast cancer. A woman must be alert to the difference—*synthetic progestogen,* not natural progesterone, was used in these studies. To date, there have been no reports of high doses of natural progesterone causing cancer in women. In fact, in her book *Once a Month*, Dr. Dalton has stated: "It is impossible to give an overdose of progesterone to a woman who has borne children, because during pregnancy women are exposed to a fifteenfold increase in their blood progesterone level for nine full months, instead of just a mere two weeks, and the body has learned to deal with that."* She writes that women who have not given birth may, with high doses of progesterone, occasionally experience menstrual cramps, or feel euphoric, or have nervous energy and be unable to sleep, but once again, these are *minor* side effects.

There is a whole range of minor side effects, or discomforts, that can be associated with progesterone use. First of all, women complain that they often have a vaginal discharge, or leakage of the suppository. To remedy this problem, a woman can cut a tampon in half, insert it into her vagina after having inserted the suppository, and lie down for ten-to fifteen-minutes. (A woman should always lie down for a ten- to fifteen-minute interval after she inserts a progesterone suppository. By remaining in a supine position for this period, she allows time for the suppository to melt, and for the body to begin absorbing the progesterone. A suppository should be inserted in the morning and in the evening.) The tampon may be removed in an hour or two. The leakage problem should be solved; however, a woman who has extensive dripping may want to use a tampon for the initial three to four hours after insertion of the progesterone.

A buildup of progesterone may cause vaginal dryness. If this is a problem, a woman may douche four hours after inserting a suppository. Also, if the dryness interferes with sexual intercourse, a woman may want to use K-Y jelly or another lubricant during lovemaking. The suppository should be inserted *after* sexual intercourse.

Many women have said they have diminished sex drive while on progesterone, and since this effect has become known, PMS patients sometimes do not want to take progesterone for fear they will have difficulty reaching orgasm. I have found that although some women report a loss of libido, others claim that, indirectly, progesterone increases sexuality because they have a general feeling of well-being and they therefore are more ready and able to enjoy lovemaking.

Progesterone also affects the normal menstrual cycle. This hormone can induce an early menses. On the other hand, progesterone can prolong menstruation and cause a heavy flow. It may also be the source of spotting or

---

*Katharina Dalton, *Once a Month* (Pomona, Calif.: Hunter House, 1979), p. 182.

heavier breakthrough bleeding in between menstrual periods. Bleeding disorders are the main progesterone-related problems. Since progesterone is rapidly excreted by the body, if a woman begins to maintain a certain progesterone level by inserting a suppository twice a day and then forgets the treatment for a day, this lapse in treatment will immediately induce her period. Also, if a woman continues her treatment beyond the day that her period is due, she will prevent the occurrence of menstruation; and if she continues progesterone treatment even longer, this prolonged hormonal supplementation will build up a thick uterine lining. Then, when she finally stops treatment, a woman might experience heavy bleeding or hemorrhaging. It is therefore important that a woman on progesterone treatment take her medication exactly according to her menstrual calendar, and coordinate it with the expected onset of her PMS symptoms.

When a woman takes progesterone for the first time, she might immediately feel hot flushes, but they will wear off in about thirty minutes. Also, her menstrual flow may change color and appear brownish. This color change occurs sometimes because bleeding has been reduced. There also may be vaginal swelling, vaginal itching, or yeast infections in the vagina. Progesterone has a tendency to change the vaginal environment. This environmental change even occurs during pregnancy, when progesterone is high and women then may also suffer vaginal infections. These vaginal side effects are due to the rise in progesterone itself, and they are not related to the type of suppository used. A woman will not find relief from these symptoms by switching to a rectal suppository.

Women on progesterone may also occasionally experience uterine cramps or nausea. Other complaints, although rare, are: oily skin and hair, irritability, nervous energy, fatigue, insomnia, euphoria, breast tenderness, body itch, diarrhea, flatulence, weight loss or gain, and heightened appetite. These minor side effects are often alleviated when progesterone doses are adjusted. Sometimes these effects are due to inappropriate doses or to the fact that the medication is not taken at scheduled times.

Some physicians have worried that progesterone might have an addictive effect on women, but this has not been my experience. I have found that after women have adapted to appropriate progesterone doses and have experienced a disappearance of PMS symptoms, they are often able to go off progesterone treatment quite easily. As long as a woman has received good counseling and knows all the facts about her condition and its treatment, she might, after a few cycles, begin to decrease and, finally, end her progesterone supplementation. After a few months of progesterone treatment, the body might readjust its hormonal fluctuations and continue to function with the hormones in balance. Months of having absorbed the needed progesterone seems to make the body systems work more efficiently. In other words, after PMS symptoms have been cured, and stress alleviated, a woman's hormonal fluctuations might normalize themselves; but a woman must continue the natural approach with good nutrition, mineral and vitamin supplementation, and methods of stress reduction.

## PROGESTERONE TREATMENT IN THE FUTURE

It is my belief that progesterone treatment in the future will be as common for PMS sufferers with a hormonal imbalance as insulin is for diabetic patients. Progesterone suppositories will, hopefully, be readily available. Progesterone might also be developed for use in other methods of administration. These methods may be: nasal spray, since the mucous membranes in the nose should be able to absorb the natural progesterone; long-acting implants into the skin; slow-releasing vaginal pessaries; or specially formulated oral tablets with which the breakdown of progesterone in the stomach is prevented.

## SPIRONOLACTONE IN THE TREATMENT OF PMS

Studies have linked PMS to an oversupply of renin, angiostensin, and aldosterone—adrenal hormones that are collectively called the aldosterone system. A new drug called spironolactone seems to be able to counterbalance the fluid retention, edema, and generally, the symptoms of PMT–H, which result from the increase of these adrenal hormones. In a study conducted at The Johns Hopkins University School of Medicine by Dr. Nelson H. Hendler, six out of seven women with PMS were freed from their symptoms after using spironolactone for three months.

Spironolactone is available by prescription in two forms—tablets containing 25 milligrams of spironolactone, and tablets containing 25 milligrams of spironolactone with 25 milligrams of hydrochlorothiazide. Spironolactone produces a diuretic effect, but it does not contribute to a loss of potassium. However, if a woman takes the combination tablet, her potassium should be monitored, because the hydrochlorothiazide may cause an excessive potassium loss. (The combination tablet is only indicated in cases of extreme edema that is not responsive to spironolactone alone, or when PMS exists along with hypertension.)

The recommended dose is one 25-milligram spironolactone tablet once or twice daily or every other day, depending on a woman's symptoms. Dosage should be specified according to the severity of each woman's syndrome, and the pill should only be taken when women are suffering from extreme water retention that does not respond to a salt-free diet alone. This medication should be started when water retention becomes apparent, and not at other times during the premenstruum. Then, spironolactone should only be used in indicated doses, because there is a warning with this drug. In animal tests to determine the drug's toxicity, spironolactone in high doses was shown to cause malignant breast and liver tumors in rats. No such side effects have been observed in humans, but still, it is wise to keep spironolactone dosage at a low level. The cancer in rats appeared after spironolactone was given in high doses over long periods; in humans this reaction is not expected since spironolactone is only given for a few days each month.

Spironolactone should not be considered a principal form of treatment. This drug is best used in combination with the natural approach, for relief of fluid retention and bloatedness. If a woman does not feel better with spironolactone, she should discontinue this medication.

## OTHER TREATMENTS ASSOCIATED WITH PMS

• *Diuretics.* Initially, many doctors thought premenstrual syndrome was due to water retention, and they prescribed diuretics to reduce swelling and breast tenderness. The diuretics caused fluid to be excreted, but they did not help women to overcome the psychological symptoms of PMS, and indeed, they even brought on symptoms such as tiredness and food cravings, which resulted because potassium was lost with body fluid.

A woman who is suffering from fluid retention due to PMS may find relief by cutting back on her salt intake and by drinking fewer liquids. Although caffeine is not recommended for women with certain PMS symptoms, a small exception may be made for diuretic purposes. A woman may have a half cup of weak coffee or tea, which sometimes acts like a diuretic. A woman on progesterone might find that her bloatedness is disappearing due to the diuretic effect of progesterone and that she does not even have to contemplate the use of diuretics.

A woman's treatment program should be individually formulated to her needs. It should always include the natural approach, and if fluid retention is one of her symptoms, it may be overcome in one of the ways mentioned above, along with the natural steps she is taking. If a woman and her doctor feel that an occasional diuretic may be helpful, a woman should be alert to any feelings of fatigue, which are signs of potassium depletion. Potassium-containing foods such as bananas, tomatoes, and orange juice should be added to her diet, and her potassium level should be monitored by her physician. If needed, potassium tablets can be purchased over the counter, or by prescription.

There are diuretics that are less potassium-depleting than others, and a woman who is going to take a diuretic may select one of these. Lasix (furosemide) and Dyrenium (triamterene) reduce buildup while they spare the body's potassium. If a woman has severe edema, she might be helped by spironolactone, as described above, but for a moderate case of fluid retention, a woman might take Lasix or Dyrenium. Lasix is available in 40-milligram tablets. One 40-milligram Laxis tablet may be taken every other day. Dyrenium may be administered in 50- or 100-milligram tablets, depending on the severity of a woman's symptoms. One Dyrenium tablet may be taken daily, or every other day. However, it is wise to remember that diuretics, although they may make a PMS sufferer feel a little better, are not cures in themselves.

• **Sleep Aids.** As mentioned in the natural approach, a woman often needs more sleep than usual during her premenstruum. Natural aids to an evening's slumber that is interrupted by PMS-induced anxiety are described in the "Sleep" section of the natural approach. If a woman tries all the natural methods of getting to sleep and she is still awake at night, then she might be helped by medication. This sleep aid is only a last resort and she should only be advised to take a mild insomnia reliever. Strong, addictive sleeping pills should be avoided. The body is especially sensitive to these heavy medications, and a woman may find that she falls prey to their addictive effects and that she is enveloped by a dark depression when she takes them.

There is a new insomnia reliever called Halcion (triazolam) available in .25- and .5-milligram tablets. This is a short-term drug that does not produce a "hangover effect" in the morning. Several airline attendants who were also PMS sufferers took Halcion and found that they were able to travel, adjust to different time schedules, sleep soundly, and awaken refreshed, while they were working to overcome their symptoms. Thus, it has been my experience that Halcion is a nonaddictive sleep aid that does not bring on unwanted psychological side effects.

• **Lithium.** Lithium has been effective in alleviating manic-depressive states in women, and studies have been done to determine whether it would work in severe premenstrual depressions, but there are no definite conclusions to report as yet. One study undertaken in 1966 by Dr. Samuel Gershon, chairman of psychiatry at Wayne State University School of Medicine in Detroit, suggests that lithium carbonate only be used in treating extreme cases of PMS, such as the syndromes exhibited by the British women who were arrested for violent crimes. Dr. Gershon did not find that lithium was valuable in treating moderate PMS symptoms.

Dr. Richard E. Shader, chairman of the department of psychiatry at Tufts University School of Medicine in Boston, also found success with lithium as a treatment for PMS sufferers whose syndromes not only prevented them from functioning normally but also damaged their interpersonal relationships. However, in a follow-up study among women with moderate PMS, lithium did not work any more effectively than a diuretic combined with a placebo. Here, though, is support for Dr. Gershon's suggestion that lithium is beneficial in extreme syndromes but not in milder, more common cases. The use of lithium as a PMS-reliever is still questionable.

• **L–Dopa.** L–Dopa is available as a prescription drug under various names, the most well-known being Laradopa (levodopa). L–Dopa is specifically used in the treatment of Parkinson's Disease, but it has been considered a possible treatment for women who suffer extreme nervousness and agitation from PMS. Dopamine, one of the brain's natural mood stabilizers, does not cross the blood/brain barrier, while L–Dopa does. L–Dopa is absorbed by the gastrointestinal tract, works on the nervous system, and eventually is converted into dopamine in the brain.

A woman who suffers from the nervousness and agitation of PMS may be helped by vitamin $B_6$, but if $B_6$ is ineffective and L–Dopa is suggested, she should immediately stop taking the vitamin. Vitamin $B_6$ inhibits the effect of L–Dopa.

There have been no studies to prove that L–Dopa works in combating PMS, and there are side effects to consider. Upper gastrointestinal bleeding might occur, and there could also be depression, nausea, and vomiting. If a woman is being treated with MAO-inhibitors for high blood pressure, she should not even be allowed to take L–Dopa.

A woman should be treated with different forms of the natural and medical approaches, and only if other treatments have been exhausted should her doctor even think about the possibility of administering such a powerful drug as L–Dopa. In fact, the drug has only been used in very rare cases. L–Dopa is not a principal form of treatment of PMS.

• **Birth Control Pills.** A healthy under-thirty-five woman who has no history of diabetes, cardiovascular or circulatory problems, and no fibroid tumors can safely take today's low-estrogen-containing birth control pill without the risks of cancer and circulatory problems that were attached to the high-estrogen pill of the sixties and early seventies. The original birth control pills, health-hazardous though they were, actually alleviated PMS symptoms because the estrogen was so strong. It was during those fledgling years of oral contraception that the pill became known as a treatment for PMS. The pill today should not be regarded in the same way.

Today's oral contraceptives are made with a combination of estrogen and progesterone, with estrogen content much lower than in the past, and the synthetic progesterone—progestogens—more powerful. However, as mentioned in the "Differences Between Natural Progesterone and Synthetic Progestogens" section of this chapter, women have often found that PMS symptoms intensified, or even occurred for the first time, when they were exposed to synthetic progestogens.

A woman who becomes fatigued, depressed, listless, or uninterested in sex while she is on the pill is experiencing symptoms related to excessive progestogen. She should consult with her doctor and request a pill with a different hormonal balance. However, even if a woman is able to adjust to a modern birth control pill, it is no longer an effective method of fighting the syndrome. Many women take the pill and have no sign of PMS, but if a woman feels the pill does not agree with her, she should stop taking it. When a sufferer stops the pill, she may find, as other women have, that she develops a case of PMS that is more intense than she ever had before. It has even happened that women who did not have premenstrual syndrome prior to taking the pill experienced the condition once they ended oral contraception.

A woman whose doctor suggests that she take the birth control pill as a treatment for her PMS should allow two months to pass so that her body can adjust to the new hormonal influx. If after two months she still feels out of sorts, she should try a pill with a different dosage or stop this medication altogether.

## PMS AND YOU

A great number of women have for years been suffering from symptoms caused by the hormonal imbalances in their bodies. Yet these women did not know how to identify their problems because they did not understand what was happening to them. And even though they knew *something* was wrong, they often suppressed their feelings and did not tell anyone what they thought, because they feared they might be ridiculed.

The women's movement, which increased awareness of the female body and showed the need for improved women's health care, freed women from their inhibitions about discussing their health problems. Women began to realize that they could help each other and themselves by sharing their health experiences with their doctors, families, friends, and co-workers. This new ability to communicate helped to educate many women to the existence of what has come to be known as premenstrual syndrome, or PMS.

Today, awareness of PMS is considered the first important step in combating the symptoms associated with the syndrome. Following awareness comes an understanding of the causes of PMS, and of the treatments that are available. The facts must be made clear. Premenstrual syndrome is neither an imaginary condition nor a real but incurable condition.

It is hoped that this book will provide extensive insights into PMS, while helping each sufferer discover ways to overcome its symptoms. With this book in hand, every woman who feels she may have premenstrual syndrome should be able to find modern counseling, and a cure.

PMS has been with us for centuries and has been the source of much suffering. I sincerely hope that PMS will soon be understood and treated by all medical professionals, recognized in the workplace, and accepted by the families and friends of women who are the unwilling victims of this monthly malady. The once-constant controversy over the existence of hypoglycemia has calmed down, and now the condition is recognized. If, like hypoglycemia, PMS could eventually be accepted without debate, we would all be able to work toward a complete elimination of this multifaceted problem.

# 6

## Where to Get Help for PMS

As PMS gains recognition, a burgeoning number of physicians and clinics are engaged in treating the syndrome. Many of the new PMS centers offer excellent counseling and treatment of PMS, but services are not all the same. A woman must realize that PMS care varies from physician to physician, and from clinic to clinic, and she would be wise to take time to evaluate a few facilities before she decides to make an appointment.

In researching the care offered to PMS sufferers by physicians and PMS centers across the country, my co-author and I have learned that prices and approaches to treatment have a wide range. One clinic might charge $300 for a one-day session; another may want *less* than $300 for over ten visits; while a physician who treats PMS in private practice may only request the normal fee for office visits. Blood tests for hormonal analyses usually cost extra. Even though treatment at a PMS center may be covered by health insurance, the bill may be high. A woman should inquire about what her particular insurance will pay for in regard to her PMS care.

It is our hope that treatment of PMS will become available for every woman from her own doctor. Physicians are in the process of gaining more knowledge about the diagnosis and treatment of PMS, and they are trying to learn from each other. On the West Coast, Dr. Guy E. Abraham, one of the foremost PMS researchers, has encouraged communication among physicians and health care experts in the Los Angeles area by forming the PMT Medical Society. This professional association holds monthly meetings at which doctors can discuss PMS cases they are treating and ask each other questions. Gynecologists, nutritionists, nurses, psychiatrists, psychologists, and dermatologists are all members of the PMT Medical Society, which became active three years ago. The birth of this society is definitely encouraging. Dr. Abraham, under the auspices of Optimox, Inc., is helping physicians across the country establish PMS centers where women may be treated according to his program for the natural approach to PMS relief. A woman might contact Optimox (address listed below) to find out if any of these centers are located in her area. However, at present, a woman with PMS may still have to travel for care.

We have looked into the services at well-known PMS centers, and talked to physicians who have emerged as leaders in PMS care. The centers (which may be referral organizations and/or treatment clinics) and physicians of sound reputation are listed below. A woman may want to consult doctors or PMS centers located near her home. Although women who live close to treatment centers logically benefit from these nearby facilities, many of the specialists at these centers are able to offer information about PMS care from doctors and centers in various parts of the country. A woman might learn about local services by contacting a center miles away.

As far as we know, the centers and doctors offering special services to PMS sufferers, listed alphabetically according to state, are:

PMS Institute
4541 North Seventh Street
Phoenix, Arizona 85014
602-279-2233

Dr. Lloyd B. Greig
9201 Sunset Boulevard, Suite 906
Los Angeles, California 90069
213-276-1151

The PMS Connection
Women's Medical Center
5985 West Pico Boulevard
Los Angeles, California 90035
213-937-0911

Dr. Lynous W. Hall
8363 Reseda Boulevard
Suite #9
Northridge, California 91324
213-993-0219

Optimox, Inc.
801 Deep Valley Drive
Rolling Hills Estates, California 90274
213-541-3096

Premenstrual Syndrome Consultants
 of Colorado
6900 West Alameda Avenue
Suite 404
Lakewood, Colorado 80226
303-922-9205

Dr. Michelle Harrison
763 Massachusetts Avenue
Cambridge, Massachusetts 02139
617-491-5800

The Premenstrual Syndrome Program, Inc.
40 Salem Street
Lynnfield, Massachusetts 01940
617-245-9585

PMS Research Foundation
P.O. Box 14574
Las Vegas, Nevada 89114
702-731-6476

North Jersey PMS Program
Drs. Michael Mandell and Allan Barbarosh
777 Union Street
Dover, New Jersey 07801
201-366-5000

PMS Medical Group
140 West End Avenue
New York, New York 10023
212-496-0449

The Premenstrual Syndrome Program, Inc.
800 Eastowne Drive
Chapel Hill, North Carolina 27514
919-493-5427

Premenstrual Syndrome Clinic
Box 3308
Duke University Medical Center
Durham, North Carolina 27710
919-684-5322

Dr. Raymond Peat
3977 Dillard Road
Eugene, Oregon 97405
503-342-3004

Focus on PMS
60 E. Township Line
Suite 306
Elkins Park, Pennsylvania 19117
215-379-4535

PMS Program
Department of Obstetrics and Gynecology
Hospital of the University of Pennsylvania
3400 Spruce Street
Philadelphia, Pennsylvania 19104
215-662-3329

Dr. Marvin R. Hyett
255 17th Street
Philadelphia, Pennsylvania 19103
215-545-4300

Dr. Edward Slotnick
Womens Renaissance Center
3900 Ford Road
Philadelphia, Pennsylvania 19131
215-879-9200

Premenstrual Syndrome Unit
Faculty Medical Practice Corporation
66 North Pauline
Memphis, Tennessee 38163
901-528-6696

Premenstrual Syndrome Program
C/2213 Medical Center North
Vanderbilt University Hospital
Nashville, Tennessee 37322
615-322-3447

The Premenstrual Syndrome Program, Inc.
2656 South Loop West
Houston, Texas 77054
713-661-6644

Premenstrual Syndrome Center
1430 North MacArthur Street
Suite 103
Irving, Texas 75061
214-721-1333

PMS Action
P.O. Box 9326
Madison, Wisconsin 53715
608-274-6688

PMS Directory
P.O. Box 8312
Madison, Wisconsin 53708

Studies into treatments for PMS are being conducted by highly qualified researchers at reputable institutions. PMS sufferers who would like to become involved in these usually no-fee experimental programs should contact the organizations listed below:

PMS Research Foundation
1318 Westgate Terrace
Chicago, Illinois 60607
312-996-5709

Dr. David R. Rubinow
National Institutes of Health
Building 10, Room 4C418
9000 Rockville Pike
Bethesda, Maryland 20205

The Depression Evaluation Service
Columbia University
Department of Psychiatry
New York State Psychiatric Institute
722 West 168th Street
New York, New York 10032
212-960-5734

The PMS Research Foundation can provide referrals and information for women in the Chicago area, just as the National Institutes of Health can help women in the greater Washington, D.C., area. Women with questions may also write to the clinic with which Dr. Katharina Dalton is affiliated: Premenstrual Syndrome Clinic, University College Hospital, London WC1, England.

In addition, university hospitals across the United States are beginning to organize clinics and support groups for the treatment of PMS. A woman might find that help is closer than she thinks. She might call the department of psychiatry, or the department of obstetrics and gynecology, at the teaching hospital or medical center in her area, and inquire about existing PMS programs.

If a woman has difficulty locating an understanding physician or PMS counselor who can compassionately care for her, she might find support and referral to a knowledgeable doctor or treatment program from her local women's health organization. Lately, a large number of women's health groups have become aware of the problems of PMS and have started to investigate the care that is offered to women in their areas. These health groups are listed below alphabetically according to state, and staff members will do their best to find relief for women who contact them:

## ARIZONA

Flagstaff Women's Resource Center
3 North Leroux Street, Rm. 201
Flagstaff, Arizona 86001                                    602-774-7353

## ARKANSAS

Mari Spehar Health Education Project
Box 545
Fayetteville, Arkansas 72701

## CALIFORNIA

Berkeley Women's Health Collective
2908 Ellsworth
Berkeley, California 94705                               415-843-6194

Chico Feminist Women's Health Center
330 Flume Street
Chico, California 95926                                  916-891-1911

Coalition for the Medical Rights of Women
1638B Haight Street
San Francisco, California 94117                          415-621-8030

DES Action
1638B Haight Street
San Francisco, California 94117                          415-621-8030

Everywoman's Clinic
A Feminist Woman's Health Center
1936 Linda Drive
Pleasant Hill, California 94523                          415-825-7900

Feminist Women's Health Center
6411 Hollywood Boulevard
Los Angeles, California 90028                            213-469-4844

Feminist Women's Health Center of Orange County
406 South Main Street
Santa Ana, California 92701                              714-972-2772

North Country Clinic for Women and Children
785 18th Street
Arcata, California 95521                                 707-822-2481

Oakland Feminist Women's Health Center
2930 McClure
Oakland, California 94609                                415-444-5676

San Francisco Women's Health Center
14 Precita Street
San Francisco, California 94110                          415-282-6999

Santa Cruz Women's Health Collective
250 Locust Street
Santa Cruz, California 95060                                    408-427-3500

Westside Women's Clinic
1711 Ocean Park Boulevard
Santa Monica, California 90405                                  213-450-2191

Womancare, A Feminist Women's Health Center
424 Pennsylvania
San Diego, California 92103                                     619-298-9352

## COLORADO

Women's Health Services
111 East Dale
Colorado Springs, Colorado 80903                               303-471-9492

## CONNECTICUT

New Moon Communications
Box 3488, Ridgeway Station
Stamford, Connecticut 06905                                     203-348-8529

Women's Health Services
19 Edwards Street
New Haven, Connecticut 06511                                    203-777-4781

## FLORIDA

Feminist Women's Health Center
540 West Brevard Street
Tallahassee, Florida 32303                                      904-224-9600

Gainesville Women's Health Center
805 Southwest 4th Avenue
Gainesville, Florida 32601                                      904-377-5055

Women's Center of Tampa, Inc.
609 de Leon
Tampa, Florida 33606                                            813-251-8629

## GEORGIA

Feminist Women's Health Center
580 14th Street, Northwest
Atlanta, Georgia 30318                                          404-874-7551

## IDAHO

Planned Parenthood
4301 Franklin Road
Boise, Idaho 83705                                    208-345-0760

## ILLINOIS

Chicago Women's Health Center
3435 North Sheffield
Chicago, Illinois 60657                               312-935-6126

Emma Goldman Women's Health Center
1628 West Belmont Avenue
Chicago, Illinois 60626                               312-528-4310

Health Evaluation and Referral Service (HERS)
1954 West Irving Park Road
Chicago, Illinois 60613                               312-248-0166

## INDIANA

Fort Wayne Women's Bureau, Inc.
P.O. Box 10554
Fort Wayne, Indiana 46853                             219-426-0023

## IOWA

Cedar Rapids Clinic for Women
86½ 16th Avenue, Southwest
Cedar Rapids, Iowa 52404                              319-365-9527

Emma Goldman Clinic for Women
715 North Dodge
Iowa City, Iowa 52240                                 319-337-2111

## KENTUCKY

Alternatives for Women
178 Walnut Street
Lexington, Kentucky 40507                             606-254-9319

## MAINE

PMS Society of Maine
P.O. Box 2632
South Portland, Maine 04106

## MASSACHUSETTS

APMS
c/o Jodi DuPuis
11 Scott Street
West Townsend, Massachusetts 01474

Boston Women's Health Book Collective
Box 192
West Somerville, Massachusetts 02144                    617-924-0271

Everywoman's Center Health Project
University of Massachusetts
Wilder Hall
Amherst, Massachusetts 01003                            413-545-0883

New Bedford Women's Center
252 County Street
New Bedford, Massachusetts 02740                        617-996-3341

The Premenstrual Syndrome Program, Inc.
40 Salem Street
Lynnfield, Massachusetts 01940                          617-245-9585

Women's Community Health Center
639 Massachusetts Avenue, Suite 210
Cambridge, Massachusetts 02139                          617-547-2302

## MICHIGAN

PMS Information and Support Group
4114 Eastman Road
Midland, Michigan 48640

Women's Crisis Center
306 North Division
Ann Arbor, Michigan 48104                               313-994-9100

Women's Health and Information Project
Box 110, Warriner Hall
Central Michigan University
Mt. Pleasant, Michigan 48858                            517-774-3762

## MINNESOTA

Elizabeth Blackwell Women's Health Center
2217 Nicolett Avenue
Minneapolis, Minnesota 55403                            612-872-1492

## MISSOURI

Women's Self-Help Center
27 North Newstead Avenue
St. Louis, Missouri 63108                314-531-2003

## MONTANA

Blue Mountain Women's Clinic
515 Kensington, Suite 24A
Missoula, Montana 59801                  406-542-0029

## NEBRASKA

Women's Resource Center
Room 116
14th and R Street
Nebraska Union
Lincoln, Nebraska 68588                  402-472-2597

## NEW HAMPSHIRE

New Hampshire Feminist Health Center
38 South Main Street
Concord, New Hampshire 03301             603-225-2739

New Hampshire Feminist Health Center
232 Court Street
Portsmouth, New Hampshire 03801          603-436-7588

## NEW MEXICO

Women's Health Services
805 Early Street
Santa Fe, New Mexico 87501               505-988-8869

## NEW YORK

Women's Counseling Project
Reid Hall
Barnard College
New York, New York 10027                 212-280-3063

Nassau County Office of Women's Services
1425 Old Country Road
Plainview, New York 11803                516-420-5101

Middle Earth Switchboard
2740 Martin
Bellemore, New York 11710                              516-826-0600

New Directions Resource Center for Women
Southampton College
Abney Peak
Southampton, New York 11968                            516-283-7898

Women's Center and Rape Crisis Center
56–58 Whitney Avenue
Binghamton, New York 13902                             607-723-3200

Women's Information Center
601 Allen Street
Syracuse, New York 13210                               315-478-4636

Feminist Healthworks
487A Hudson Street
New York, New York 10014                               212-929-7886

Health House
555 North Country Road
St. James, New York 11780                              516-862-6743

PMS
209-213 Middle Neck Road
Great Neck, New York 11021                             516-773-3960

Reproductive Rights National Network
17 Murray Street
New York, New York 10007                               212-267-8891

## NORTH CAROLINA

Durham Women's Center
YWCA
312 East Umstead Street
Durham, North Carolina 27707                           919-286-1258

Durham Women's Health Co-op
YWCA
809 Proctor Street
Durham, North Carolina 27707                           919-688-4396

## OHIO

Planned Parenthood of Summit County
39 East Market
Akron, Ohio 44308                                        216-535-2671

Project Woman
712 North Fountain
Springfield, Ohio 45504                                  513-325-3707

Womanspace
1258 Euclid Avenue #200
Cleveland, Ohio 44115                                    216-696-6967

## OKLAHOMA

Women's Treatment Center
1309 East 35 Place
Tulsa, Oklahoma 74105                                    918-749-0828

## OREGON

Portland Women's Health Center
6510 Southeast Foster
Portland, Oregon 97206                                   503-777-7044

## PENNSYLVANIA

Women's Center and Shelter of Greater Pittsburgh
P.O. Box 5147
Pittsburgh, Pennsylvania 15206                           412-661-6066

Women's Resource Center, Inc.
312–15A Bank Towers Building
Spruce Street and Wyoming Avenue
Scranton, Pennsylvania 18503                             717-346-4671

Centre County Women's Resource Center
111 Sowers Street, Suite 210
State College, Pennsylvania 16801                        814-234-5222

Lackawanna County Medical Society
1416 Monroe Avenue
Dunmore, Pennsylvania 18509                              717-344-3616

Elizabeth Blackwell Health Center for Women
112 South 16th Street
Philadelphia, Pennsylvania 19102                         215-563-7577

## RHODE ISLAND

Rhode Island Women's Health Collective
2 Stimson Avenue
Providence, Rhode Island 02906                    401-274-9264

## SOUTH DAKOTA

Brookings Women's Center
802 11th Avenue
Brookings, South Dakota 57006                    605-688-4518

## TEXAS

The Austin Women's Center
1505 West 6th
Austin, Texas 78703                    512-472-1990

PMS Support Group of Dallas/Fort Worth
3417 Cardinal Lane
Irving, Texas 75062                    214-255-9616

## UTAH

Birth and Family Center
291 W. 5400 S.
Murray, Utah 84107                    801-261-5585

Phoenix Institute
383 S. 600 E.
Salt Lake City, Utah 84102                    801-532-5080

Rocky Mountain PMS Society
P.O. Box 11314
Salt Lake City, Utah 84116                    801-355-4673

## VERMONT

Southern Vermont Women's Health Center
187 North Main Street
Rutland, Vermont 05701                    802-775-1946

Vermont Women's Health Center
336 North Avenue
Burlington, Vermont 05401                    802-863-1386

## VIRGINIA

Williamsburg Area Women's Center
P.O. Box 126
Williamsburg, Virginia 23185                                    804-229-7944

## WASHINGTON

Acadia
1827 12th Avenue
Seattle, Washington 98122                                        206-323-9388

Elizabeth Blackwell Women's Clinic
203 West Holly Street
Bellingham, Washington 98225                                     206-734-8592

Fremont Women's Clinic
6817 Greenwood Avenue, North
Seattle, Washington 98103                                        206-789-0773

Olympia Women's Center for Health
410 South Washington
Olympia, Washington 98501                                        206-943-6924

Yakima Feminist Women's Health Center
2002 Englewood, Suite B
Yakima, Washington 98902                                         509-575-6422

## WASHINGTON, D.C.

Washington Women's Self-Help
P.O. Box 1604
Washington, D.C. 20013                                           202-462-3224

## WISCONSIN

Bread and Roses Women's Health Center
238 West Wisconsin Avenue, Suite 700
Milwaukee, Wisconsin 53203                                       414-278-0260

PMS Action
P.O. Box 9326
Madison, Wisconsin 53715                                         608-274-6688

# 7

# Bibliography

PMS has been around a long time. It is amazing that doctors have appeared confused when their patients have asked them about the condition, since so many researchers have published extensive findings about it. Premenstrual syndrome has been the subject of more than three hundred scientific articles, which have been used as references for this book.

My co-author and I have compiled a bibliography that includes over three hundred articles, from leading national and international medical journals, and books that explore premenstrual syndrome. It is clear from this list of sources that a description of PMS and its treatment was presented more than fifty years ago by Dr. Robert T. Frank, a distinguished physician at Mount Sinai Medical School in New York. Since then, researchers have continued to support his contention that PMS is real. Today, as the bibliography shows, an extensive body of evidence proves that PMS is not imaginary.

This bibliography is meant to be used as a resource for women who want to know more about their conditions, as well as for their doctors. Any medical library should have the listed articles, and a reading of past PMS studies might be able to help a woman and her physician understand the condition more fully. Today we are really focusing on a revival of an old problem that for religious and political reasons could not be discussed before. Now we can speak out, and with freer communication in the future, the list of over three hundred articles should expand to such a high number that there can be no more doubt that we have fully researched and finally conquered this "imaginary disease."

A few books listed in the bibliography are excellent starting points from which women may begin their PMS educations. Particularly noteworthy are Dr. Katharina Dalton's two books: *Once a Month* and *The Premenstrual Syndrome and Progesterone Therapy.* Other books such as *The Curse,* by Janice Delaney, Mary Jane Lupton, and Emily Toth (E. P. Dutton, New York, 1976), and *Menstruation and Menopause,* by Paula Weideger (Knopf, New York, 1976), describe the dilemmas women faced before PMS became a reality.

This bibliography aims to help a woman and her physician become equal partners who work together toward a common goal—victory over PMS.

## BIBLIOGRAPHY

Abraham, G. 1981. Premenstrual tension. In *Current Problems in Obstetrics and Gynecology,* pp.1–39. Chicago: Yearbook Medical Publishers.

Abraham, G., and Hargrove, J. 1980. Effect of vitamin $B_6$ on premenstrual symptomatology in women with premenstrual tension syndrome: A double-blind crossover study. *Infertility* 3:155.

Abramson, M., and Torghele, J. R. 1961. Weight, temperature changes, and psychosomatic symptomatology in relation to the menstrual cycle. *Am. J. Obstet. Gynecol.* 81:223.

Adams, P. W.; Rose, D. P.; Folkard, J.; Wynn, V.; Seed, M.; and Strong, R. 1973. Effect of pyridoxine hydrochloride (vitamin $B_6$) upon depression associated with oral contraception. *Lancet* 1:897.

Adams, P. W.; Wynn, V.; Seed, M.; and Folkard, J. 1974. Vitamin $B_6$, depression and oral contraception. *Lancet* 2:516.

Adler, R. A.; Noel, G. I.; Wartolsky, L.; and Frantz, A. G. 1974. Failure of oral water loading and intravenous hypotonic saline to suppress plasma prolactin in man. *J. Clin. Endocrinol. Metab.* 41:383.

Adolphe, A. B.; Dorsey, E. R.; and Napoliello, M. J. 1977. The neuropharmacology of depression. *Dis. Neurol. Syst.* 38:841.

Alexander, R. W.; Gill, J. R.; Yamabe, H.; Lovenberg, W.; and Keiser, H. R. 1974. Effects of dietary sodium and of acute saline infusion on the interrelationship between dopamine excretion and adrenergic activity in man. *J. Clin. Invest.* 54:194.

Allen, E., and Doisey, E. A. 1923. An ovarian hormone: A preliminary report on its localization, extraction and partial purification and action in test animals. *J. Am. Med. Assoc.* 81:819.

Andersch, B.; Abrahamsson, L.; Wendestam, C.; Ohman, R.; and Hahn, L. 1979. Hormone profile in premenstrual tension: Effects of bromocriptine and diuretics. *Clin. Endocrinol.* 11:657.

Andersch, B.; Hahn, L.; and Isaksson, B. 1978. Body water and weight in patients with premenstrual tension. *Br. J. Obstet. Gynaecol.* 85:546.

Andersch, B.; Hahn, L.; Wendestam, C.; Ohman, R.; and Abrahamsson, L. 1978. Treatment of premenstrual tension syndrome with bromocryptine. *Acta. Endocrinol.* (Suppl. 88) 216:165.

Andersen, A. N.; Larsen, J. F.; Steenstrup, O. R.; Svendstrup, B.; and Nielsen, J. 1977. Effect of bromocriptine on the premenstrual syndrome. A double-blind clinical trial. *Br. J. Obstet. Gynaecol.* 81:370.

Appleby, B. P. 1960. A study of premenstrual tension in general practice. *Br. Med. J.* 1:391.

Argonz, J., and Abinzano, C. 1950. Premenstrual tension treated with vitamin A. *J. Clin. Endocrinol. Metab.* 10:1579.

Assaykeen, T. A., and Ganong, W. F. 1971. The sympathetic nervous system and renin secretion. In *Frontiers in Neuroendocrinology,* eds. L. Martini and W. F. Ganong, pp. 67–102. London, Ontario, Canada: Oxford University Press.

Asscher, A. W., and Jones, J. H. 1965. Capillary permeability to plasma proteins. *Postgrad. Med. J.* 41:425.

Backstrom, T., and Carstensen, H. 1974. Estrogen and progesterone in plasma in relation to premenstrual tension. *J. Steriod. Biochem.* 5:257.

Backstrom, T., and Mattsson, B. 1975. Correlation of symptoms in premenstrual tension to oestrogen and progesterone concentrations in blood plasma. *Neuropsychobiology* 1:80.

Baden, W. F., and Lizcano, H. R. 1964. Evaluation of a new diuretic drug (Quinethazone) in the premenstrual tension syndrome. *J. New Drugs* 3:167.

Ball, S. G., and Lee, M. R. 1977. The effect of carbidopa administration on urinary sodium excretion in man. Is dopamine an intrarenal natriuretic hormone? *Br. J. Clin. Pharmacol.* 4:115.

Barry, V. C., and Klawans, H. L. 1976. On the role of dopamine in the pathophysiology of anorexia nervosa. *J. Neural Transm.* 38:107.

Baumann, G., and Loriaux, D. L. 1976. Failure of endogenous prolactin to alter renal salt and water excretion and adrenal function in man. *J. Clin. Endocrinol. Metab.* 43:643.

Baumann, G.; Marynick, S. P.; Winters, S. J.; and Loriaux, D. L. 1977. The effect of osmotic stimuli on prolactin secretion and renal water excretion in normal man and in chronic hyperprolactinemia. *J. Clin. Endocrinol. Metab.* 44:199.

Behrman, S. J. 1961. Premenstrual tension. *Am. J. Obstet. Gynecol.* 81:606.

Benedek-Jaszmann, L. J., and Hearn-Sturtevant, M. D. 1976. Premenstrual tension and functional infertility. *Lancet* 1:1095.

Berger, I. L. 1955. Ulcerative stomatitis caused by endogenous progesterone. *Ann. Intern. Med.* 42:205.

Bergland, R. M., and Page, R. B. 1979. Pituitary-brain vascular relations: A new patadigm. *Science* 204:18.

Berl, T.; Brautbar, N.; Ben-David, M.; Czaczkes, W.; and Kleeman, D. 1976.Osmotic control of prolactin release and its effect on renal water excretion in man. *Kidney Int.* 10:158.

Bickers, W., and Woods, M. 1951. Premenstrual tension—rational treatment. *Tex. Rep. Biol. Med.* 9:406.

Bierman, S. M. 1973. Autoimmune progesterone dermatitis of pregnancy. *Arch. Dermatol.* 107:896.

Billig, H. F., and Spaulding, C. A. 1947. Hyperinsulinism of menses. *Indust. Med.* 16:336.

Biskind, M. 1943. Nutritional deficiency in the etiology of menorrhagia, metrorrhagia, cystic mastitis and premenstrual tension: treatment with vitamin B complex. *J. Clin. Endocrinol. Metab.* 3:227.

Biskind, M. S., and Biskind, G. R. 1942. Effect of vitamin B complex deficiency on inactivation of estrone in the liver. *Endocrinology* 31:109.

———. 1943. Inactivation of testosterone propionate in the liver during vitamin B complex deficiency. Alteration of the estrogen-androgen equilibrium. *Endocrinology* 32:97.

Biskind, M. S.; Biskind, G. R; and Biskind, L. H. 1944. Nutritional deficiency in the etiology of menorrhagia, metrorrhagia, cystic mastitis and premenstrual tension. *Surg. Gynecol. Obstet.* 78:49.

Bisset, G. W.; Chowdrey, H. S.; and Feldberg, W. 1978. Release of vasopressin by enkephalin. *Br. J. Pharmacol.* 62:370.

Bjorklund, A.; Moore, R. Y.; Nobin, A.; and Stenevi, U. 1973. The organization of tuberohypophyseal and reticulo-infundibular catecholamine neuron systems in the rat brain. *Brain Res.* 51:171.

Block, E. 1960. The use of vitamin A in premenstrual tension. *Acta. Obset. Gynecol. Scand.* 39:585.

Bond, G. C.; Pasley, J. N.; Koike, T. I.; and Llerna, L. 1976. Contamination of an ovine prolactin preparation with antidiuretic hormone. *J. Endocrinol.* 71:169.

Bridges, T. E.; Hillhouse, E. W.; and Jones, M. T. 1976. The effect of dopamine on neurohypophyseal hormone release in vivo and from the rat neural lobe and hypothalamus in vitro. *J. Physiol.* 260:647.

Briggs, M., and Briggs, M. 1972. Relationship between monoamine oxidase activity and sex hormone concentration in human blood plasma. *J. Reprod. Fertil.* 29:447.

Brown, J. D., and Doe, R. P. 1978. Pituitary pigmentary hormones. Relationship of melanocyte stimulating hormone to lipotropic hormone. *JAMA* 240:1274.

Brown, D. R., and Holtzman, S. G. 1979. Suppression of deprivation-induced food and water intake in rats and mice by naloxone. *Pharmacol. Biochem. Behav.* 11:567.

Brown, J. J.; Davies, D. L.; Lever, A. F.; and Robertson, J. L. S. 1964. Variations in plasma renin during the menstrual cycle. *Br. Med. J.* 2:1114.

Bruce, J., and Russell, G. F. M. 1962. Premenstrual tension—a study of weight changes and balances of water, sodium, and potassium. *Lancet* 2:267.

Bryant, G. D., and Greenwood, F. C. 1971. In *Lactogenic Hormones,* eds. G. E. W. Wolstenholme and J. Knight, p. 202. London: Churchill Livingstone.

Buckman, M. T.; Kaminsky, N.; Conway, M.; and Peake, G. T. 1973. Utility of L-dopa and water loading in evaluation of hyperprolactinemia. *J. Clin. Endocrinol. Metab.* 36:911.

Buckman, M. T., and Peake, G. T. 1973. Osmolar control of prolactin secretions in man. *Science* 181:755.

Canales, F. S., Sotia, J.; Zarate, A.; Mason, M.; and Molina, M. 1976. The influence of pyridoxine on prolactin secretion and milk production in women. *Br. J. Obstet. Gynaecol.* 83:387.

Carey, R. M., and Johanson, A. J. Prolactin-induced antidiuresis in man. In Abstracts of The Endocrine Society Annual Meeting, Baltimore, 1976, The Williams & Wilkins Co. (Abst. No. 216).

Carey, R. M.; Thorner, M. O.; and Ortt, E. M. 1979. Effects of metaclopramide and bromocryptine on the renin-angiotensin-aldosterone system in man: do-paminergic control of aldosterone. *J. Clin. Invest.* 63:727.

Carlsson, A., and Lindquist, M. 1973. Effect of ethanol on the hydroxylation of tyrosine and tryptophan in the rat brain in vivo. *J. Pharm. Pharmacol.* 25:437.

Carroll, B., and Steiner, M. 1978. The psychobiology of premenstrual dysphoria: the role of prolactin. *Psychoneuroendocrinology.* 3:171.

Celis, F. 1977. Effect of estrogen and progesterone on the release of MSH in gonadectromized rats. *Neuroendocrinology* 24:119.

Chau-Pham, T. T. 1978. The opiate receptors and the discovery of opioid-like peptides. *Drug Metab. Rev.* 7:255.

Chiorboli, E., and Miller dePaiva, L. 1966. Excretion of aldosterone in premenstrual tension. *Arq. Bras. Endocrinol. Metab.* 15:107.

Clark, D.; Thody, A. J.; Shuster, S.; and Bowers, H. 1978. Immunoreactive a-MSH in human plasma in pregnancy. *Nature* 273:163.

Cole, E. N.; Everend, D.; Horrobin, D. F.; Manku, M. S.; Miabaji, J. P.; and Nassar, B. A. 1975. Is prolactin a fluid and electrolyte regulating hormone in man? *J. Physiol.* 25:54.

Collier, H. O. J., and Roy, A. C. 1974. Morphine-like drugs inhibit the stimulation by E prostaglandins of cyclic AMP formation by rat brain homogenates. *Nature* 248:24.

Coppen, A., and Kessel, N. 1963. Menstruation and personality. *Br. J. Psychiatry* 109:711.

Corner, G. W., and Allen, W. M. 1929. Physiology of the corpus luteum. II. Production of a special uterine reaction (progestational proliferation) in response to the corpus luteum. *Am. J. Physiology* 88:326.

Cort, J. H.; Cort, J.; Navakova, J.; and Skopkova, J. 1974. Interaction of vasopressins and linear N-terminal ACTH fragments in the induction of natriuresis. *Eur. J. Clin. Invest.* 4:293.

Costovsky, R.; Wajchenberg, B. I.; and Nogneira, O. 1974. Hyperresponsiveness to lysine-vasopressin in Cushing's disease. *Acta. Endocrinol.* 75:125.

Coupar, I. M. 1978. Inhibition by morphine of prostaglandin stimulated fluid secretion in rat jejunum. *Br. J. Pharmacol.* 63:57.

Craig, P. E. 1953. Premenstrual tension and the menopause. *Med. Times* 81:485.

Crane, M. G.; Heitsch, J.; Harris, J. J.; and Johns, V. J., Jr. 1966. Effect of ethinyl estradiol (Estinyl) on plasma renin activity. *J. Clin. Endocrinol. Metab.* 26:1403.

Creutzfeldt, W. 1973. Gastrointestnal hormones and insulin secretion. *N. Engl. J. Med.* 288:1238.

Crowley, W. R.; O'Donahue, T. L.; George, J. M.; and Jacobowitz, D. M. 1978. Changes in pituitary oxytocin and vasopressin during the estrous cycle and after ovarian hormones: Evidence for mediation by norepinephrine. *Life Sci.* 23:2579.

Cuche, J. L.; Kuchel, O.; Barbeau, A.; Boucher, R.; and Genest, J. 1972. Relationship between the adrenergic nervous system and renin during adaption to upright posture: A possible role for dopamine. *Clin. Sci.* 43:481.

Cullberg, J. 1972. Mood changes and menstrual symptoms with different estrogen combinations. *Acta. Psychiatr. Scand.* (Suppl.) 236:1.

Dalton, K. 1960. Effect of menstruation on schoolgirls' weekly work. *Br. Med. J.* 1:326.

———. 1960. Menstruation and accidents. *Br. Med. J.* 2:1425.

———. 1961. Menstruation and crime. *Br. Med. J.* 2:1752.

Dalton, K. 1965. The influence of menstruation on health and disease. *Proc. R. Soc. Med.* 57:18.

―――. 1977. *The Premenstrual Syndrome and Progesterone Therapy.* London: William Heinemann Medical Books Ltd.

―――. 1979. *Once a Month. The Premenstrual Syndrome: What It is and How to Free Yourself from its Effects.* Pomona, California: Hunter House.

Danforth, D. N.; Boyer, P. K.; and Graff, S. 1946. Fluctuation in weight, hematocrit and plasma protein with the menstrual cycle. *Endocrinology* 39:188.

Davidson, J. M. 1978. Gonadal hormones and human behavior. In *Hormonal Contraceptives, Estrogens and Human Welfare,* eds. M. D. Diamond and C. G. Korenbrot, pp. 127–128. New York: Academic Press.

De Fronzo, R.; Deibert, D.; Hendler, R.; Felig, P.; and Soman, V. 1979. Insulin sensitivity and insulin binding to monocytes in maturity-onset diabetes. *J. Clin. Invest.* 63:939.

Delitala, G.; Masala, A.; Alagna, S.; and Devilla, L. 1978. Effect of pyridoxine on human hypophyseal trophic hormone release: A possible stimulation of hypothalamic dopaminergic pathway. *J. Clin. Endocrinol. Metab.* 42:293.

DePirro, R.; Fusco, A.; Bertoli, A.; Greco, A. V.; and Lauro, R. 1978. Insulin receptors during the menstrual cycle in normal women. *J. Clin. Endocrinol. Metab.* 47:1387.

DeWaal, J. M.; Steyn, A. P.; Harms, J. H. K.; Slabber, C. F.; and Pannall, P. R. 1978. Failure of pyridoxine to suppress raised serum prolactin levels. *S. Afr. Med.* 53:293.

Edeiken, J., and Griffith, J. Q., Jr. 1940. Cyclic pulmonary edema at menses in mitral stenosis. *JAMA* 115:287.

Edwards, C. R. W.; Besser, G.; and Thorner, M. D. 1979. Bromocryptine-responsive form of idiopathic edema. *Lancet* 2:94.

Edwards, O. M., and Bayliss, R. I. S. 1973. Urinary excretion of water and electrolytes in normal females during the follicular and luteal phases of the menstrual cycle: The effect of posture. *Clin. Sci.* 45:495.

Ehara, Y.; Siler, T.; VandenBerg, G.; Sinha, Y. N.; and Yen, S. S. C. 1973. Circulating prolactin levels during the menstrual cycle: Episodic release and diurnal variation. *Am. J. Obstet. Gynecol.* 117:962.

Ellinwood, E. H.; Sudilovsky, A.; and Nelson, L. M. 1973. Evolving behavior in the clinical and experimental amphetamine (model) phychosis. *Am. J. Psychiatry* 130:1088.

Elsner, C.; Buster, J.; Schindler, R. et al. 1980. Bromocryptine in the treatment of premenstrual tension syndrome. *Obstet. Gynecol.* 56:723.

Epstein, M. T.; Hockaday, J. M.; and Hockaday, T. D. R. 1978. Migraine and reproductive hormones throughout the menstrual cycle. *Lancet* 1:543.

Epstein, S.; van Zyl-Smit, R.; LeRoith, D.; Vinik, A.; and Pimstone, B. 1977. The effects of TRH on prolactin, plasma renin activity, water and electrolyte excretion in normal males. *Horm. Metab. Res.* 9:496.

Ernest, E. M. 1961. Preliminary clinical report on trichlormethiazide in premenstrual tension. *Curr. Ther. Res.* 3:221.

Farah, F. S., and Shbaklu, A. 1971. Autoimmune progesterone urticaria. *J. Allergy Clin. Immunol* 48:257.

Faucheux, B.; Buu, N. T.; and Kuchel, O. 1977. Effects of saline and albumin on plasma and urinary catecholamines in dogs. *Am. J. Physiol.* 232:123.

Ferris, T. F.; Chonko, A. M.; Williams, J. S.; Reineck, H. J.; and Stein, J. H. 1973. Studies of the mechanism of sodium retention in idiopathic edema. *Trans. Assoc. Am. Physicians* 86:310.

Fitzsimmons, J. T. 1978. Angiotensin, thirst and sodium apppetite: retrospect and prospect. *Fed. Proc.* 37:2609.

Fitzsimmons, J. T.; Kucharczyk, J.; and Richards, G. 1978. Systemic angiotensin induced drinking in the dog: A physiological phenomenon. *J. Physiol.* (London) 276:435.

Fitzsimmons, J. T., and Setler, P. E. 1975. The relative importance of central nervous catecholaminergic and cholinergic mechanisms in drinking in response to angiotensin and other thirst stimuli. *J. Physiol.* (London) 250:613.

Fortin, J. N.; Wittkower, E. D.; and Kalz, F. 1958. A psychosomatic approach to the premenstrual tension syndrome. A preliminary report. *Can. Med. Assoc. J.* 79:978.

Foukas, M. D. 1973. An antilactogenic effect of pyridoxine. *Br. J. Obstet. Gynaecol.* 80:718.

Franchimont, P.; Dourey, C.; Legros, J. J.; Reuter, A.; Vrindts-Gevaert, Y.; Van Cauwenberge, J. R.; and Gaspard, U. 1976. Prolactin levels during the menstrual cycle. *Clin. Endocrinol.* (Oxford) 5:643.

Frank, M. M.; Gelfand, J. A.; and Atkinson, J. P. 1976. Hereditary angioedema: The clinical syndrome and its management. *Ann. Intern. Med.* 84:580.

Frank, R. T. 1931. The hormonal causes of premenstrual tension. *Arch. Neurol. Psychiatry* 26:1053.

Fregly, M. J. 1978. Attenuation of thirst in estrogen-treated rats. *Fed. Proc.* 37:2694.

Fuxe, K.; Lofstrom, A.; Hokfelt, T.; Ferland, L.; Andersson, K.; Agnati, L.; Eneroth, P.; Gustafsson, J.; and Skett, P. 1978. Influence of central catecholamines on LHRH containing pathways. *Clin. Obstet. Gynecol.* 5:251.

Geiringer, E. 1951. A reconsideration of premenstrual phenomena. *Br. J. Obstet. Gynaecol.* 58:1010.

Gerber, J. 1939. Desensitization in the treatment of menstrual intoxication and other allergic symptoms. *Br. J. Dermatol.* 51:265.

Gerber, J. 1921. Einiges zur Pathologic der Urticaria menstruals. *Dermatol. Z.* 32:143.

Ghose, K., and Coppen, A. 1977. Bromocryptine and premenstrual syndrome: controlled study. *Br. Med. J.* 1:147.

Gianutsos, G., and Lal, H. 1978. Narcotic analgesics and aggression. *Mod. Probl. Pharmacopsychiatry* 13:114.

Glass, G. S.; Heninger, G. R.; Lansky, M.; and Talan, K. 1971. Psychiatric emergency related to the menstrual cycle. *Am. J. Psychiatry* 128:705.

Goldberg, L. T. 1972. Cardiovascular and renal actions of dopamine: Potential clinical applications. *Pharmacol. Rev.* 24:1.

Goldberg, L. T.; McDonald, R. H. Jr.; and Zimmerman, A. M. 1963. Sodium diuresis produced by dopamine in patient with congestive heart failure. *N. Engl. J. Med.* 269:1060.

Goldzieher, J. W.; Moses, L. E.; Averkin, E.; Scheel, C.; and Taber, B. F. 1971. Nervousness and depression attributed to oral contraceptives: A double-blind, placebo-controlled study. *Am. J. Obstet. Gynecol.* 111:1013.

Golub, L. J.; Menduke, H.; and Conley, S. S. 1965. Weight changes in college women during the menstrual cycle. *Am. J. Obstet. Gynecol.* 91:89.

Graham, J. J.; Harding, P. E.; Wise, P. H.; and Berriman, H. 1978. Prolactin suppression in the treatment of premenstrual syndrome. *Med. J. Aust.* (Suppl.) 2:18.

Grandison, L., and Guidotti, A. 1977. Stimulation of food intake by muscimol and Beta endorphin. *Neuropharmacology* 16:533.

Grant, L. D., and Stumpf, W. 1975. Hormone uptake sites in relation to central nervous system biogenic amine systems. *Anatomical Neuroendocrinology,* pp. 445–463. Basel: S. Karger A. G.

Gray, L. A. 1941. The use of progesterone in nervous tension states. *South. Med. J.* 34:1004.

Gray, M. J.; Strausfled, K. S.; Watanabe, M.; Sims, E. A. H.; and Solomon, S. 1968. Aldosterone secretory rates in the normal menstrual cycle. *J. Clin. Endocrinol. Metab.* 28:1269.

Greenblatt, R. B. 1940. Syndrome of major menstrual molimina with hypermenor-rhea alleviated by testosterone propionate. *JAMA* 115:120.

Greene, R., and Dalton, K. 1953. The premenstrual syndrome. *Br. Med. J.* 1:1007.

Greenhill, J. P., and Freed, S. C. 1941. The electrolyte therapy of premenstrual distress. *JAMA* 117:504.

———. 1940. The mechanism and treatment of premenstrual distress with ammonium chloride. *Endocrinol.* 26:529, 1940.

Halbreich, U.; Ben-David, M.; Assael, M.; and Bornstein, R. 1976. Serum-prolactin in women with premenstrual syndrome. *Lancet* 2:654.

Hargrove, J., and Abraham, G. 1979. Effect of vitamin $B_6$ on infertility in women with the premenstrual tension syndrome. *Infertility* 2:315.

———. 1981. Endocrine profile of patients with post-tubal ligation syndrome. *J. Reprod. Med.* 26:359.

———. 1982. The incidence of premenstrual tension in a gynecologic clinic. *J. Reprod. Med.* 27:721.

Harris, S. 1944. Hyperinsulinism. *South. Med. J.* 37:711.

Hays, R. M. 1976. Antidiuretic hormone. *N. Engl. J. Med.* 295:659.

Hays, R. M., and Levine, S. D. 1974. Vasopressin. *Kidney Int.* 6:307.

Heckel, G. P. 1953. Endocrine allergy and the therapeutic use of pregnanediol. *Am. J. Obstet. Gynecol.* 66:1297.

———. 1951. Endogenous allergy to steroid hormones. *Surg. Gynecol. Obstet.* 92:191.

———. 1949. The problem of allergy to steroid hormones. *J. Clin. Endocrinol. Metab.* 9:681.

Heckel, G. P., and Scherp, H. W. 1955. Allergenic properties of pregnanediol. *J. Clin. Endocrinol. Metab.* 15:877.

Hendler N. 1980. Spironolactone for premenstrual syndrome. *The Female Patient* 5:17.

Herzberg, B. N. 1971. Body composition and premenstrual tension. *J.Psychosom. Res.* 15:251.

Herzberg, B., and Coppen, A. 1970. Changes in psychological symptoms in women taking oral contraceptives. *Br. J. Psychiatry* 116:161.

Herzberg, B. N.; Draper, K. C.; Johnson, A. L.; and Nicol, G. C. 1971. Oral contraceptive, depression and libido. *Br. Med. J.* 1:495.

Herzberg, B. N., Johnson, A. L.; and Brown, S. 1970. Depressive symptoms and oral contraceptives. *Br. Med. J.* 4:142.

Hodge, R. L.; Lowe, R. C.; and Vane, J. R. 1966. The effects of alteration of blood volume on the concentration of circulating angiotensin in anaesthetized dogs. *J. Physiol.* 186:613.

Holtzman, S. G. 1975. Effects of narcotic antagonists on fluid intake in the rat. *Life Sci.* 16:1465.

Horrobin, D. F.; Lloyd, I. J.; Lipton, A.; Burstyn, P. G.; Durkin, N.; and Muiruri, K. L. 1971. Actions of prolactin on human renal function. *Lancet* 2:352.

Howe, A., and Thody, A. J. 1970. The effect of ingestion of hypertonic saline on the melanocyte stimulating hormone content of the pars intermedia of the rat pituitary gland. *J. Endocrinol.* 46:201.

Husami, N.; Idriss, W.; Jewelewicz, R.; Ferin, M.; and Vande Wiele, R. L. 1978. Lack of acute effects of pyridoxine on prolactin secretion and lactation. *Fertil. Steril.* 30:393.

Interim report from the oral contraception study of the Royal College of General Practitioners. London, 1974. Sir Isaac Pitman & Sons, Ltd., p. 29.

Ipp, E.; Dobbs, R.; and Unger, R. H. 1978. Morphine and B-endorphin influence the secretion of the endocrine pancreas. *Nature* 276:190.

Israel, S. L. 1938. Premenstrual tension. *JAMA* 110:1721.

Ivey, M. E., and Bardwick, J. M. 1968. Patterns of affective fluctuation in the menstrual cycle. *Psychosom. Med.* 30:336.

Iwamoto, E. T., and Way, E. L. 1979. Opiate actions and catecholamines. *Adv. Biochem. Psychopharmacol.* 20:357.

Janowsky, D. S.; Berens, S. C.; and Davis, J. M. 1973. Correlations between mood, weight and electrolytes during the menstrual cycle: A renin-angiotensin-aldosterone hypothesis of premenstrual tension. *Psychosom. Med.* 35:143.

Jarrett, R. J., and Graver, H. J. 1968. Changes in oral glucose tolerance during the menstrual cycle. *Br. Med. J.* 2:528.

Johnson, J. A.; Davis, J. O.; Baumber, J. S.; and Schneider, E. G. 1970. Effects of estrogens and progesterone on electrolyte balances in normal dogs. *Am. J. Physiol.* 219:1691.

Jones, E. M.; Fox, R. H.; Verow, P. W.; and Asscher, A. W. 1966. Variations in capillary permeability to plasma proteins during the menstrual cycle. *Br. J. Obstet. Gynaecol.* 73:666.

Jones, W. N., and Gordon, V. H. 1969. Autoimmune progesterone eczema—an endogenous progesterone hypersensitivity. *Arch. Dermatol.* 99:57.

Jordheim, O. 1972. The premenstrual syndrome. *Acta. Obstet. Gynecol. Scand.* 51:77.

————. 1972. The premenstrual syndrome: Clinical trials of treatment with a progestogen combined with a diuretic compared with both a progestogen alone and with a placebo. *Acta. Obstet. Gynecol. Scand.* 51:77.

Judd, S., and McMurdo, R. 1976. The premenstrual syndrome. *Mod Med.* (Aust.) 19:16.

Jung, Y.; Khurana, R. C.; Corredor, D. G.; Hastillo, A.; Lain, R. F.; Patrick, D.; Turkeltaub, P.; and Danowski, T. S. 1971. Reactive hypoglycemia in women. *Diabetes* 20:428.

Jungck, E. C.; Barfield, W. E.; and Greenblatt, R. B. 1952. Chlorothiazide and premenstrual tension. *JAMA* 169:96.

Katz, F. H., and Kappas, A. 1967. The effects of estradiol and estriol on plasma levels of cortisol and thyroid hormone-binding globulins and on aldosterone and cortisol secretion rates in man. *J. Clin. Invest.* 46:1768.

Katz, F. H., and Romth, P. 1972. Plasma aldosterone and renin activity during the menstrual cycle. *J. Clin. Endocrinol. Metab.* 34:819.

Kaulhausen, H.; Leyendecker, G.; Beuker, A.; and Breuer, H. 1978. The relationship of the renin-angiotensin-aldosterone system to plasma gonadotropin, prolactin and ovarian steroid patterns during the menstrual cycle. *Arch. Gynecol.* 225:179.

Kerr, G. D. 1977. The management of the premenstrual syndrome. *Curr. Med. Res. Opin.* 4:29.

Kincl, F. A.; Ciaccio, L. A.; and Benagiano, G. 1978. Increasing oral bio-availability of progesterone by formulation. *J. Ster. Biochem.* 9:83.

Klaiber, E.; Kobayashi, Y.; Broverman, D.; et al. 1971. Plasma monoamine oxiduse activity in regularly menstruating women and in amenorrheic women receiving cyclic treatment with estrogens and progesten. *J. Clin. Endocrinol.* 33:630.

Klein, L., and Carey, J. 1957. Total exchangeable sodium in the menstrual cycle. *Am. J. Obstet. Gynecol.* 74:956.

Korossy, S. 1975. Autoimmune progesterone urticaria and dermatitis. In *Immunological Aspects of Allergy and Allergic Diseases,* vol. 3, eds. S. Korossy and E. Raijka, pp. 154–155. New York: Plenum.

Kuchel, O.; Buu, N. T.; and Unger, T. 1978. Dopamine sodium relationship. Is dopamine a part of the endogenous natriuretic system? *Contrib. Nephrol.* 13:27.

Kuchel, O.; Cuche, J. L.; Buu, N. T.; Guthrie, G. P.; Unger, P.; Nowaczvuski, W.; Boucher, R.; and Genest, J. 1977. Catecholamine excretion in "idiopathic" edema decreased dopamine excretion. A pathogenic factor. *J. Clin. Endocrinol. Metab.* 44:639.

Kuchel, O.; Hamet, P.; Cuche, J. L.; Polis, G.; Fraysse, J.; and Gehest, J. 1975. Urinary and plasma cyclic adenosine $3'.5'$-monophosphate in patients with idiopathic edema. *J. Clin. Endocrinol. Metab.* 41:282.

Kuchel, O.; Horky, K.; Gregorova, I.; Marek, J.; Kopecka, J.; and Kobilkova, J. 1970. Inappropriate response to upright posture: A precipitating factor in the pathogenesis of idiopathic edema. *Ann. Intern. Med.* 73:245.

Kupperman, H. S. 1963. Dysmenorrhea and premenstrual molimina. In *Human Endocrinology,* pp. 356–383. Philadelphia: F. A. Davis Co.

Kurtman, N. A., and Boonjarern, S. 1975. Physiology of antidiuretic hormone and the interrelationship between the hormone and the kidney. *Nephron.* 15:167–185.

Kutner, S. J., and Brown, W. L. 1972. Types of oral contraceptives, depression and premenstrual symptoms. *J. Nerv. Ment. Dis.* 155:153.

Lal, H., and Puri, S. K. 1972. Morphine withdrawal aggression: role of dopaminergic stimulation. In *Drug Addiction: Experimental Pharmacology,* eds. J. M. Singh, L. Miller, and H. Lal, p. 301. Mount Kisco, New York: Futura Publishing Co.

Lamb, W. M., Ulett, G. A.; Masters, W. H.; and Robinson, D. 1953. Premenstrual tension: FEG, hormonal and psychiatric evaluation. *Am. J. Psychiatry* 109:810.

Landau, R. L., and Lugibihl, K. 1958. Inhibition of the sodium-retaining influence of aldosterone by progesterone. *J. Clin. Endocrinol. Metab.* 18:1237.

―――. 1961. The catabolic and natriuretic effects of progesterone in man. *Recent Prog. Horm. Res.* 17:219.

Lauersen, N. H., and Graves, Z. R. 1983. A new approach to premenstrual syndrome. *The Female Patient,* 8:41.

Lauersen, N. H., and Stukane, E. 1982. *Listen to Your Body. A Gynecologist Answers Women's Most Intimate Questions.* New York: Simon & Shuster.

Lauersen, N. H., and Wilson, K. H. 1977. Evaluation of danazol as an oral contraceptive. *Obstet. Gynecol.* 50:91.

―――. 1976. The effects of danazol in the treatment of chronic cystic mastitis. *Obstet. Gynecol.* 43:93.

Lauersen, N. H.; Wilson, K. H.; and Birnbaum, S. 1975. Danazol: an antigonadotropic agent in the treatment of pelvic endometriosis. *Am. J. Obstet. Gynecol.* 123:742.

Layne, D.; Meyer, C. J.; Vaishwaner, P. S.; and Pincus, G. 1962. The secretion and metabolism of cortisol and aldosterone in normal and in steroid-treated women. *J. Clin. Endocrinol. Metab.* 22:107.

Lebtovirta, P.; Tanta, T.; and Seppala, M. 1978. Pyridoxine treatment of galactorrhea-amenorrhea syndromes. *Acta. Endocrinol.* 87:682.

Legros, J. J.; Gilot, P.; Seron, N.; Claessens, J.; Adam, A.; Moeglen, J. M.; Audibert, A.; and Berchier, P. 1978. Influence of vasopressin on learning and memory. *Lancet* 1:11.

Lichtensteiger, W., and Lienhart, R. 1977. Response of mesencephalic and hypothalamic dopaminergic neuroses to a-MSH: Mediated by area postrema? *Nature* 266:635.

Liebowitz, M. R., and Klein, D. F. 1979. Hysteroid Dysphoria. *Psych. Clin. N. Am.* 2:555.

Lightman, S. L.; and Forsling, M. L. 1980. Evidence for endogenous opioid control of vasopressin release in man. *J. Clin. Endocrinol. Metab.* 50:569.

Lloyd, C. W. 1964. Problems associated with the menstrual cycle. In *Human Reproduction and Sexual Behaviour,* ed. C. E. Lloyd, pp. 291–295. Philadelphia: Lea & Febiger.

Lorame, J. A., and Bell, E. T. 1971. In *Hormone Assays and Their Clinical Application,* pp. 408–409. Baltimore: Williams & Wilkins.

MacDonald, H. N.; Collins, Y. D.; Tobin, M. J. W.; and Wijavaratne, D. N. 1976. *Br. J. Obstet. Gynaecol.* 83:54.

McDonald, R. H. Jr., Goldberg, L. L.; McNay, J. L.; and Tuttle, E. P. Jr. 1961. Effects of dopamine in man: Augmentation of sodium excretion glomerular filtration rate and renal plasma flow. *J. Clin. Invest.* 43:1116.

McGuinness, B. W. 1961. Skin pigmentation and the menstrual cycle. *Br. Med. J.* 2:563.

McIntosh, E. N. 1976. Treatment of women with galactorrhea-amenorrhea syndrome with pyridoxine (vitamin $B_6$). *J. Clin. Endocrinol. Metab.* 42:1192.

McIntyre, N.; Holdsworth, C. D.; and Turner, D. S. 1965. Intestinal factors in the control of insulin secretion. *J. Clin. Endocrinol. Metab.* 25:1317.

Malarkey, W. B.; George, J. M.; and Baehler, R. W. 1975. Evidence for vasopressin contamination of ovine and bovine prolactin. *Int. Res. Commun. Syst.* 3:291.

Marcus, R. G. 1975. Suppression of lactation with high dose of pyridoxine. *S. Afr. Med. J.* 49:2155.

Mata, M.; Gainer, H.; and Klee, W. A. 1977. Effect of dehydration on the endogenous opiate content of the rat neurointermediate lobe. *Life Sci.* 21:1159.

Mattsson, B., and Schoultz, B. V. 1974. A comparison between lithium, placebo and a diuretic in premenstrual tension. *Acta. Psychiatr. Scan.* (Suppl.) 225:75.

Means, E., and Grant, E. C. G. 1962. "Anoular" as an oral contraceptive. *Br. Med. J.* 2:75.

Michelakis, A. M.; Stant, E. G.; and Brill, A. B. 1971. Sodium space and electrolyte excretion during the menstrual cycle. *Am. J. Obstet. Gynecol.* 109:150.

Michelakis, A. M.; Yoshida, H.; an Dormois, J. C. 1975. Plasma renin activity and plasma aldosterone during the normal menstrual cycle. *Am. J. Obstet. Gynecol.* 123:724.

Miller, L. H.; Kastin, A. J.; Sandman, C. A.; Fink, M.; and Vanveen, W. J. 1974. Polypeptide influences on attention, memory and anxiety in man. *Pharmacol. Biochem. Behav.* 2:663.

Miller, M., and Wilks, J. W. 1973. Urinary antidiuretic hormone excretion during the menstrual cycle and pregnancy in the monkey. *Neuroendocrinology* 12:174.

Miller, R. J., and Cuatrecasas, P. 1978. Enkephalins and endorphins. *Vitam. Horm.* 36:297.

Milligan, D.; Drife, J.O.; and Short, R. V. 1975. Changes in breast volume during normal menstrual cycle and after oral contraceptives. *Br. Med. J.* 4:494.

Moo's, R. H. 1968. Psychological aspects of oral contraceptives. *Arch. Gen. Psychiatry* 19:87.

Morgan, C. M., and Hadley, M. E. 1976. Ergot alkaloid inhibition of melanophore stimulating hormone secretion. *Neuroendocrinology* 21:10.

Morley, J. E. 1980. The neuroendocrine control of appetite: The role of endogenous opiates, cholecystokinin, TRH, gamma amino-butyric-acid and the diazepam receptor. *Life Sci.* 27:355.

Morris, M. N., and Udry, J. R. 1972. Contraceptive pills and day-by-day feelings of well being. *Am. J. Obstet. Gynecol.* 113:763.

Morton, J. H. 1950. Premenstrual tension. *Am. J. Obstet. Gynecol.* 60:343.

———. 1953. Treatment of premenstrual tension. *Int. Rec. Med.* 166:505.

Morton, J. H.; Addition, H.; Addison, R. G.; Hunt, L.; and Sullivan, J. J. 1953. A clinical study of premenstrual tension. *Am. J. Obstet. Gynecol.* 65:1182.

Mosonyi, L. 1975. The role of the neuroendocrine system in immunopathological processes. In *Immunological aspects of allergy and allergic diseases,* eds. E. Rajka and S. Korossy, vol. 6, pp. 81–118. New York: Plenum.

Mukherjee, C. 1954. Premenstrual tension. A critical study of the syndrome. *J. Ind. Med. Assoc.* 24:81.

Munday, M.; Brush, M. G.; and Taylor, R. W. 1977. Progesterone and aldosterone levels in premenstrual tension syndrome. *J. Endocrinol.* 73:21P.

Negoro, H.; Visessuwan, S.; and Holland, R. C. 1973. Unit activity in the paraventricular nucleus of female rats at different stages of the reproductive cycle and after ovariectomy, with or without estrogen or progesterone treatment. *J. Endocrinol.* 95:545.

Nemeroff, C. B., and Prauge, A. J., Jr. 1978. Peptides and psychoneuroendocrinology. *Arch. Gen. Psychiatry* 35:999.

Nillius, S. J., and Johansson, E. D. B. 1971. Plasma levels of progesterone after vaginal, rectal, or intramuscular administration of progesterone. *Am. J. Obstet. Gynecol.* 110: 470.

Nilson, L.; and Solvell, L. 1962. Clinical studies on oral contraceptives—a randomized double-blind crossover study of four different preparations. *Acta. Obstet. Gynecol. Scand.* (Suppl. 8) 46:1.

Nilsson, A.; Jacobson, L.; and Ingemanson, C. A. 1967. Side effects of an oral contraceptive with particular attention to mental symptoms and sexual adaptation. *Acta. Obstet. Gynecol. Scand.* 46:537.

Nokin, J.; Vekemans, M.; and Robyn, C. Circadian periodicity of serum prolactin concentration in man. *Br. Med. J.* 3:561.

Noth, R. H.; McCallum, R. W.; Contino, C.; and Havelick, J. 1980. Tonic dopaminergic suppression of plasma aldosterone. *J. Clin. Endocrinol. Metabol.* 51:61.

Oelkers, W.; Schonesholer, M.; and Blumel, A. 1974. Effects of progesterone and four synthetic progestogens on sodium balance and the renin-aldosterone system in man. *J. Clin. Endocrinol. Metab.* 39:882.

O'Donohue, T. L.; Miller, R. L.; Pendleton, R. C.; and Jacobowitz, D. M. 1979. A diurnal rhythm of immunoreactive a-melanocyte stimulating hormone in discrete regions of the rat brain. *Neuroendocrinology* 29:281.

Okey, R., and Robb, E. L. 1925. Studies of the metabolism of women. I. Variations in the fasting blood sugar level and in sugar tolerance in relation to the menstrual cycle. *J. Biol. Chem.* 65:165.

Okey, R.; and Stewart, D. 1932–33. Diet and blood cholesterol in normal women. *J. Biol. Chem.* 99:717.

Oparil, S.; Ehrlich, E. N., and Lindheimer, M. D. 1975. Effect of progesterone on renal sodium handling in man. Relation to aldosterone excretion and plasma renin activity. *Clin. Sci.* 49:139.

Ostfeld, A. M. Studies in headache: Migraine and the menstrual cycle. In *Psychosomatic Obstetrics, Gynaecology and Endocrinology,* ed. W. S. Kroger, pp. 327–333. Springfield, Illinois: Charles C. Thomas.

Pagani, C. 1952. Tensione premenstruale, e vitamina A. *Acta. Vitaminol. Enzymol.* (Milano) 6:24.

Paldino, R. L., and Hyman, C. 1954. Mechanism whereby renin increases the rate of T-1824 disappearance from the circulation of rabbits. *Am. J. Physiol.* 179:599.

Parker, A. S. 1960. The premenstrual tension syndrome. *Med. Clin. North Am.* 44:339.

Paulson, M. J. 1961. Psychological concomitants of premenstrual tension. *Am. J. Obstet. Gynecol.* 81:733.

Peart, W. S. 1978. Renin: 1978. *Johns Hopkins Med. J.* 143:193.

Pennington, V. M. 1957. Meprobamate in premenstrual tension. *JAMA* 164:638.

Penny, R. J.; Tilders, F. J. H.; and Thody, A. J. 1979. The role of dopaminergic tuberohypophysial neurons in the maintenance of basal melanocyte stimulating hormone levels in the rat. *J. Endocrinol.* 80:58P.

Perr, I. N. 1958. Medical, psychiatric and legal aspects of premenstrual tension. *Am. J. Psychiatry* 115:211.

Perrini, A.; and Piliego, N. 1959. The increases of aldosterone in the premenstrual syndrome. *Minerva Med.* 50:2897.

Peters, F.; Zimmermann, G.; and Breckwoldt, M. 1978. Effect of pyridoxine on plasma levels of HGH, PRL and TSH in normal women. *Acta. Endocrinol.* 89:217.

Petersen, W. F., and Milles, G. 1926. The relation of menstruation to the permeability of the skin capillaries and the autonomic tonus of the skin vessels. *Arch. Intern. Med.* 38:730.

Piliego, N.; Rossini, P.; Del Zotti, G.; and Scardapane, R. 1964. Gli effetti di un carico di follicolina sull'aldosteronuria e sulla catecolaminuria di donne normali e con sindrome premestruale. *Folia Endocrinol.* 17:391.

Preece, P. E.; Richards, A. R.; Owen, G. M.; and Hughes, L. F. 1975. Mastalgia and total body water. *Br. Med. J.* 4:498.

Preedy, J. R. K., and Aitken, F. H. 1956. The effect of estrogen on water and electrolyte metabolism. I. The normal. *J. Clin. Invest.* 35:423.

Quigley, M. E., and Yen, S. S. C. 1980. The role of endogenous opiates on LH secretion during the menstrual cycle. *J. Clin. Endocrinol. Metab.* 51:179.

Ramsay, D. J.; Reid, J. A.; Keil, L. C.; and Ganong, W. F. 1978. Evidence that the effects of isoproterenol on water intake and vasopressin secretion are mediated by angiotensin. *Endocrinology* 103:54.

Reed, J. L., and Ghodse, A. H. 1973. Oral glucose tolerance and hormonal response in heroin-dependent males. *Br. Med. J.* 2:582.

Rees, L. 1953. Psychosomatic aspects of the premenstrual tension syndrome. *J. Ment. Sci.* 99:62.

———. 1953. The premenstrual tension syndrome and its treatment. *Br. Med. J.* 1:1014.

Reich, M. 1962. The variations in urinary aldosterone levels of normal females during their menstrual cycle. *Aust. Ann. Med.* 11:41.

Reid, R. L., Hoff, J. D., Yen, S. C. C., and Li, C. H. 1980. Effects on pituitary hormone secretion and disappearance rate of exogenous Bh-endorphin in normal human subjects. *J. Clin. Endocrinol. Metab.*

Reid, R. L.; Ling, N.; and Yen, S. S. C. In press. Amelanocyte stimulating hormone induces gonadotropin release. *J. Clin. Endocrinol. Metab.*

Reid, R. L., and Yen, S. S. C. B-Endorphin stimulates the secretion of insulin and glucagon in humans. In preparation.

———. 1981. Premenstrual Syndrome. *Am. J. Obstet. Gynecol.* 139:86.

Rennick, B. R. 1968. Dopamine: renal tubular transport in the dog and plasma binding studies. *Am. J. Physiol.* 215:532.

Roberts, J. S., and Share, L. 1970. Inhibition by progesterone of oxytocin secrection during vaginal stimulation. *Endocrinology* 87:812.

Robertson, G. L. 1974. Vasopressin in osmotic regulation in man. *Annu. Rev. Med.* 23:315.

Rogers, W. C. 1962. The role of endocrine allergy in the production of premenstrual tension. *West. J. Surg. Obstet. Gynecol.* 70:100.

Ropert, J. F., and Yen, S. S. C. In press. Endogenous opiates modulate pulsatile LH release in humans. *J. Clin. Endocrinol. Metab.*

Rose, D. P. 1978. The interactions between vitamin $B_6$ and hormones. *Vitam. Horm.* 36:53.

Roy, S. K.; Ghosh, B. P.; and Blattacharjee, S. K. 1971. Changes in oral glucose tolerance during normal menstrual cycle. *J. Indian Med. Assoc.* 57:201.

Ruble, D. N. 1977. Premenstrual symptoms: A reinterpretation. *Science* 197:291.

Sampson, G. A. 1979. Premenstrual syndrome: A double-blind controlled trial of progesterone and placebo. *Brit. J. Psychiat.* 135:209.

Scheiner, F. 1975. The relationship of antidiuretic hormone to the control of volume and tonicity in the human. *Adv. Clin. Chem.* 17:1.

Schmid, F. 1953. L'évolution de la glycémie chez le chien morphinisé chroniquement. *C. R. Soc. Bio.* (Paris) 147:129.

Schwartz, J. C.; Pollar, C.; Llorens, B.; Malfroy, C.; Gros, P.; Pradelle, S.; and Dray, F. 1978. Endorphins and endorphin receptors in the striatum: relationships with dopaminergic neurons. *Adv. Biochem. Psychopharmacol.* 18:245.

Schwartz, U., and Abraham, G. 1975. Corticosterone and aldosterone levels during the menstrual cycle. *Obstet. Gynecol.* 45:339.

Seeman, P., and Lee, T. 1974. The dopamine releasing actions of neuroleptics and ethanol. *J. Pharmacol. Exp. Ther.* 190:131.

Sellers, A. L.; Smith, S.; Marmorston, J.; and Goodman, H. C. 1952. Studies of the mechanism of experimental proteinuria. *J. Exp. Med.* 96:643.

Severs, W. B., and Summy-Long, J. 1975. The role of angiotensin in thirst. *Life Sci.* 17:1513.

Shabanah, E. H. 1963. Treatment of premenstrual tension. *Obstet. Gynecol.* 21:49.

Shangold, M. M. 1982. PMS is real, but what can you do about it? *Contemp. OB/ GYN* 19:251.

Shelley, W. B.; Preucel, R. W., and Spoont, S. S. 1964. Autoimmune progesterone dermatitis—cure by oophorectomy. *JAMA* 190:147.

Simantov, R., and Snyder, S. H. 1977. Optate receptor binding in the pituitary gland. *Brain Res.* 124:178.

Simkin, B., and Arce, R. 1963. Prolactin activity in blood during the normal human menstrual cycle. *Proc. Soc. Exp. Biol. Med.* 113:485.

Simkins, S. 1947. Use of massive doses of vitamin A in the treatment of hyperthyroidism. *J. Clin. Endocrinol. Metab.* 7:572.

Simmons, R. J. 1956. Premenstrual tension. *Obstet. Gynecol.* 8:99.

Singer, K.; Cheung, R.; and Schon, M. 1974. A controlled evaluation of lithium in the premenstrual tension syndrome. *Br. J. Psychiatry* 124:50.

Skinner, S. L.; Lumbers, F. R.; and Symonds, E. M. 1969. Alteration by oral contraceptives of normal menstrual changes in plasma renin activity, concentration and substrate. *J. Clin. Sci.* 36:67.

Skowsky, R., and Swan, L. Androgen and estrogen regulation of arginine vasopressin in the castrate male and female rat: Evidence for pituitary feedback, presented at Endocrine Society Meeting, Anaheim, Calif., 1979, p. 161 (Abst. No. 355).

Sletten, T. W., and Gershon, S. 1966. The premenstrual syndrome: A discussion of its pathophysiology and treatment with lithium ion. *Compr. Psychiatry* 7:197.

Smith, S. L. 1976. The menstrual cycle and mood disturbance. *Clin. Obstet. Gynecol.* 19:391.

Snyder, S. H. 1977. Opiate receptors and internal opiates. *Science* 236:44.

Sofroniew, M. U., and Weindle, A. 1978. Projections from the parvocellular vasopressin and neurophysin containing neurons of the suprachiasmatic nucleus. *Am. J. Anat.* 153:391.

Somerville, B. W. 1971. The role of progesterone in menstrual migraine. *Neurology* 21:853.

Sommer, B. 1972. Menstrual cycle changes and intellectual performance. *Psychosom. Med.* 34:263.

Spellacy, W. N.; Carlson, K. I.; and Schade, S. L. 1967. Menstrual cycle carbohydrate metabolism. *Am. J. Obstet. Gynecol.* 99:382.

Stieglitz, E., and Kimble, S. 1949. Premenstrual intoxication. *Am. J. Med. Sci.* 218:616.

Suarez-Murias, E. L. 1953. The psychophysiologic syndrome of premenstrual tension with emphasis on the psychiatric aspect. *Int. Rec. Med.* 166:475.

Sundsfjord, J. A., and Aakvaag, A. 1970. Plasma angiotensin H and aldosterone excretion during the menstrual cycle. *Acta. Endocrinol.* 64:152.

———. 1972. Plasma renin activity, plasma renin substrate and urinary aldostetone excretion in the menstrual cycle in relation to the concentration of progesterone and oestrogens in the plasma. *Acta. Endocrinol.* 71:519.

Sutherland, H., and Steward, I. 1965. A critical analysis of the premenstrual syndrome. *Lancet* 2:1180.

Taggart, N. 1962. Diet, activity and body weight. A study of variations in a woman. *Br. J. Nutr.* 16:223.

Taleisnik, S., and Tomatis, M. E. 1969. Effect of estrogen on pituitary melanocyte-stimulating hormone content. *Neuroendocrinology* 5:24.

———. 1970. Mechanisms that determine the changes in Pituitary MSH activity during pseudopregnancy induced by vaginal stimulation in the rat. *Neuroendocrinology* 6:368.

Taylor, R. W. 1977. The treatment of premenstrual tension with dydrogesterone. *Curr. Med. Res. Opin.* 4:35–10.

Thody, A. J. 1977. The significance of melanocyte-stimulating hormone (MSH) and the control of its secretion in the mammal. *Adv. Drug Res.* 11:23.

Thody, A. J., and Shuster, S. 1973. Possible role of FSH in the mammal. *Nature* 245:207.

Thomas, W. A. 1933. Generalized edema occurring only at the menstrual period. *JAMA* 101:1126.

Thorn, G. W., and Engel, L. L. 1938. The effect of sex hormones on the renal excretion of electrolytes. *J. Exp. Med.* 68:299.

Thorn, G. W.; Nelson, K. R.; and Thorn, D. W. 1938. A study of the mechanism of edema associated with menstruation. *Endocrinology* 22:155.

Timonen, S., and Procope, B. 1971. Premenstrual syndrome and physical exercise. *Acta. Obstet. Gynecol. Scand.* 50:331.

Tolis, G.; Laliberte, R.; Guyda, H.; and Naftolin, F. 1977. Ineffectiveness of pyridoxine ($B_6$) to alter secretion of growth hormone and prolactin and absence of therapeutic effects on galactorrhea-amenorrhea syndromes. *J. Clin. Endocrinol. Metab.* 44:1197.

Urbach, F. 1939. Menstruation allergy. *New Int. Clin.* 2:160.

Vander, A. J., and Geelhoed, G. W. 1965. Inhibition of renin secretion by angiotensin II. *Proc. Soc. Exp. Biol. Med.* 120:399.

Van Praag, H. M. 1978. Neuroendocrine disorders in depression and their significance for the monoamine hypothesis of depression. *Acta. Psychiatr. Scand.* 57:389.

Van Vugt, D. A., and Meites, J. 1980. Influence of endogenous opiates on anterior pituitary function. *Fed. Proc.* 39:2533.

Vainder, M. 1951. Theory and rationale in the treatment of premenstrual tension and dysmenorrhea. *Indust. Med. Surg.* 20:199.

Veit, H. 1955. Psychosomatic aspects of premenstrual tension. *Wis. Med. J.* 54:599.

Vekeman, M.; Delvoye, P.; L'Hermite, M.; and Robyn, C. 1977. Serum prolactin levels during the menstrual cycle. *J. Clin. Endocrinol Metab.* 44:989.

Venning, E. H.; Dyrenfurth, I.; and Beck, J. C. 1957. Effect of anxiety upon aldosterone excretion in man. *J. Clin. Endocrinol. Metab.* 17:1005.

Vigersky, R. A.; Andersen, A. E.; Thompson, R. H.; and Loriaux, D. L. 1977. Hypothalamic dysfunction in secondary amenorrhea associated with simple weight loss. *N. Engl. J. Med.* 297:1141.

Vivas, A., and Celis, M. 1978. Differences in the release of melanocyte-stimulating hormone in vitro by rat pituitary glands collected at various times during the oestrous cycle. *J. Endocrinol.* 78:1.

Von Klein, H. O. 1954. Vitamin-A-therapie bei pramenstruellen nervösen beschwerden. *Disch. Med. Wochenschr.* 79:879.

Vorherr, H.; Vorherr, U. F.; and Solomon, S. 1978. Contamination of prolactin preparations by antidiuretic hormone and oxytocin. *Am. J. Physiol.* 234:F318.

Vuolteenaho, O.; Vakkuri, O.; and Leppaluoto, J. 1980. Wide distribution of B-endorphin-like immunoreactivity in extrapituitary tissues of rat. *Life Sci.* 27:57.

Watson, P. E., and Robinson, M. F. 1965. Variations in body weight of young women during the menstrual cycle. *Br. J. Nutr.* 19:237.

Wei, F., and Loh, H. 1976. Physical dependence on opiate-like peptides. *Science* 193:1262.

Weitzman, R. E.; Fisher, D. A.; Minick, S.; Ling, N.; and Guillemin, R. 1977. B-endorphin stimulates secretion of vasopressin in vivo. *Endocrinology* 101:1643.

Wetzel, R. D.; Reich, T.; McClure, J. N.; and Wald, J. A. 1975. Premenstrual affective syndrome and affective disorder. *Br. J. Psychiatry* 127:219.

Whitehead, M. I.; Townsend, P. T.; Gill, D. K.; Collins, W. P.; and Campbell, S. Absorption and metabolism of oral progesterone. *Brit. Med. J.* 825–827.

Widholm, O.; Frisk, M.; Tenhunen, T.; and Hartling, H. 1967. Gynecological findings in adolescence: A study of 514 patients. *Acta. Obstet. Gynecol. Scand.* (Suppl. 10) 46:10.

Wilkes, M. M.; Watkins, W. B.; Stewart, R. D.; and Yen, S. S. C. 1980. Localization and quantitation of B-endorphin in human brain and pituitary. *Neuroendocrinology* 30:113.

Wilson, C. A. 1974. Hypothalamic amines and the release of gonadotrophins and other anterior pituitary hormones. *Adv. Drug. Res.* 8:119.

Wolny, H. L.; Plech, A.; and Herman, A. S. 1974. Diuretic effects of intraventricularly injected noradrenaline and dopamine in rats. *Experientia* 30:1062.

Wong, W. H.; Freedman, R. I.; Levan, N. E.; Human, C.; and Quilligan, F. J. 1972. Changes in the capillary filtration coefficient of cutaneous vessels in women with premenstrual tension. *Am. J. Obstet. Gynecol.* 114:950.

Zeppa, R. 1969. Vascular response of the breast to estrogens. *J. Clin. Endocrinol. Metab.* 29:695.

Zimmerman, F. A.; Carmel, P. W.; Husain, M. K.; Ferin, M.; Tannenbaum, M.; Frantz, A. G.; and Robinson, A. G. 1973. Vasopressin and neurophysin: High concentrations in monkey hypophyseal portal blood. *Science* 182:925.

Ziserman, A. J. 1935. Ulcerative vulvitis and stomatitis of endocrine origin. *JAMA* 104:826.

Zondek, B., and Bromberg, Y. M. 1947. Clinical reactions of allergy to endogenous hormones and their treatment. *Br. J. Obstet. Gynaecol.* 54:1.

———. 1945. Endocrine allergy. *J. Allergy Clin. Immunol.* 16:1.

Zondek, B., and Brezezinski, A. 1948. Inactivation of oestrogenic hormone by women with vitamin B deficiency. *Br. J. Obstet. Gynaecol.* 55:273.

*Menstrual Calendar:* Mark your symptoms, as explained in Chapter 4, on this calendar. Note if your symptoms worsen on or around the onset of menstruation. Symptoms should be marked for 2 to 3 months so that you may see if they appear in a regular, cyclic pattern. There should be a symptom-free interval each month for PMS to exist.

# MENSTRUAL CALENDAR

| DAY: | MONTH: | MONTH: | MONTH: |
|---|---|---|---|
| 1 | | | |
| 2 | | | |
| 3 | | | |
| 4 | | | |
| 5 | | | |
| 6 | | | |
| 7 | | | |
| 8 | | | |
| 9 | | | |
| 10 | | | |
| 11 | | | |
| 12 | | | |
| 13 | | | |
| 14 | | | |
| 15 | | | |
| 16 | | | |
| 17 | | | |
| 18 | | | |
| 19 | | | |
| 20 | | | |
| 21 | | | |
| 22 | | | |
| 23 | | | |
| 24 | | | |
| 25 | | | |
| 26 | | | |
| 27 | | | |
| 28 | | | |
| 29 | | | |
| 30 | | | |
| 31 | | | |

# MENSTRUAL CALENDAR

| DAY: | MONTH: | MONTH: | MONTH: |
|------|--------|--------|--------|
| 1 | | | |
| 2 | | | |
| 3 | | | |
| 4 | | | |
| 5 | | | |
| 6 | | | |
| 7 | | | |
| 8 | | | |
| 9 | | | |
| 10 | | | |
| 11 | | | |
| 12 | | | |
| 13 | | | |
| 14 | | | |
| 15 | | | |
| 16 | | | |
| 17 | | | |
| 18 | | | |
| 19 | | | |
| 20 | | | |
| 21 | | | |
| 22 | | | |
| 23 | | | |
| 24 | | | |
| 25 | | | |
| 26 | | | |
| 27 | | | |
| 28 | | | |
| 29 | | | |
| 30 | | | |
| 31 | | | |

# MENSTRUAL CALENDAR

| DAY: | MONTH: | MONTH: | MONTH: |
|---|---|---|---|
| 1 | | | |
| 2 | | | |
| 3 | | | |
| 4 | | | |
| 5 | | | |
| 6 | | | |
| 7 | | | |
| 8 | | | |
| 9 | | | |
| 10 | | | |
| 11 | | | |
| 12 | | | |
| 13 | | | |
| 14 | | | |
| 15 | | | |
| 16 | | | |
| 17 | | | |
| 18 | | | |
| 19 | | | |
| 20 | | | |
| 21 | | | |
| 22 | | | |
| 23 | | | |
| 24 | | | |
| 25 | | | |
| 26 | | | |
| 27 | | | |
| 28 | | | |
| 29 | | | |
| 30 | | | |
| 31 | | | |

# MENSTRUAL CALENDAR

| DAY: | MONTH: | MONTH: | MONTH: |
|---|---|---|---|
| 1 | | | |
| 2 | | | |
| 3 | | | |
| 4 | | | |
| 5 | | | |
| 6 | | | |
| 7 | | | |
| 8 | | | |
| 9 | | | |
| 10 | | | |
| 11 | | | |
| 12 | | | |
| 13 | | | |
| 14 | | | |
| 15 | | | |
| 16 | | | |
| 17 | | | |
| 18 | | | |
| 19 | | | |
| 20 | | | |
| 21 | | | |
| 22 | | | |
| 23 | | | |
| 24 | | | |
| 25 | | | |
| 26 | | | |
| 27 | | | |
| 28 | | | |
| 29 | | | |
| 30 | | | |
| 31 | | | |

# Index

abdomen, 104, 138, 162, 172
  cramps in, 86, 165
  swelling of, 17, 44, 72, 117-118, 123
abortion, 98
Abraham, Guy E., 43-46, 120, 156, 184-185
*acini*, 104
Adams, P. W., 41
adrenal hormones (aldosterone system), 45,
  70-71, 119, 170, 178
adrenalin, 72, 134, 163
age, 60-61, 88
agitation as symptom, 17, 36, 62, 63, 119,
  122, 124, 132, 159, 163
alcohol, 124-125, 167
alcoholism, 115
aldosterone, 45, 70-71, 119, 178
aldosterone system, 70-71, 119, 178
alpha-melanocyte-stimulating-hormone
  (alpha-MSH), 54
amenorrhea, 54, 57, 165
*American Journal of Obstetrics and Gynecol-
  ogy,* 53
amino acids, 54, 64, 123
ammonium chloride, 40
ammonium nitrate, 40
amphetamines, 66
Anaprox (naproxen sodium), 84-85, 161
androstenedione, 59-60
anemia, 57, 68, 107, 130
angiotensin, 70, 178
Ann, 80-81
anorexia nervosa, 98
antidepressants, 157, 159
antiprostaglandins, 160-161
anxiety, 36, 44, 117-118, 128, 153, 166
*Archives of General Psychiatry,* 124
*Archives of Neurology and Psychiatry,* 34
Armour Thyroid, 164
aspirin, 84, 160, 161
asthma, 17, 22, 36, 42, 168

backache, 17
basal body temperatures (BBTs), 29-30,
  99-100, 101, 106

Beauvoir, Simone de, 33
Benson, Stephanie, 27
beta-endorphin, 54
Bible, 22
Bickers, William, 38, 40
birth control pills, 41, 67, 72-73, 98, 102,
  132, 169, 175, 181-182
Biskind, Morton S., 40-41
bloatedness, 17, 40, 44, 62, 72, 80, 123,
  128, 130, 152, 156, 179
  *see also* water retention
blood tests, 107-108, 110, 111, 117, 166,
  167, 172
brain, 58-59, 123, 181
brain hormones, 46, 52, 53-54, 59, 75, 118,
  120, 122, 163
breakfast, PMS dietary, 126
breast cancer, 70, 170
breast disease, fibrocystic (FBD), 104, 134,
  162-163
breast tenderness, 17, 36, 72, 80, 92, 104,
  165, 177, 179
breathing, rhythmic, 140-141
*British Journal of Psychiatry,* 171
Brody, Jane, 121
bromocriptine, 71-72, 132, 160, 165
Brush, M. G., 136

caffeine, 123, 155
calcium, 56, 88, 108, 128-129, 130, 134,
  135, 158
calcium gluconate tablets, 128-129
cancer, 76, 134, 158, 170, 175
*Carbohydrate Craver's Diet, The* (Wurtman),
  64, 122
carbohydrates, 61, 120-123, 126, 127, 167
  natural, 121
carotene, 134
catecholamines, 72
CBC (Complete Blood Count), 107
cervix, 83, 85, 106, 158
Chaorati, 30
cholesterol, 60, 136, 168
collagen, 134

**219**

19183